Praise for *MenoWars*

'This brilliant book provides a fascinating overview of how we have reached the current state of confusion over menopause management, where medical misinformation and over-commercialisation are rife, leaving women unsure of who and what to believe. Fiona tackles the issues with wit and science, giving us her personal experiences as well as evidence-based advice from trusted medical experts.'

– **Dr Juliet Balfour**, GP and BMS-accredited menopause specialist

'Fiona Clark has achieved the impossible; an engaging and interesting book on menopause that breaks down the myths in a relatable, conversational style, while incorporating the best scientific data. In an environment that is saturated with influencers and advice, Fiona Clark's career as an investigative journalist shines through – she writes with credibility and authority; no stone is left unturned.'

– **Suzanne Smith**, Australian award-winning investigative journalist and author of *The Altar Boys*

'The menosphere is currently a chaotic, confusing and sadly messy space, and women are feeling more confused, overwhelmed and conflicted than ever before. That's why books like this are so important. As a highly experienced and well-regarded science journalist and editor, you can be reassured that everything Fiona writes will be fact-checked, impartial and evidence-based. I recommend that every woman, man, health care and media professional devour this book!'

– **Katie Taylor**, founder of The Latte Lounge and author of *Midlife Matters*

'Nothing like a smart, savvy Australian to tell it like it is – Fiona delivers an evidence-based, myth-busting, badass take on menopause that finally answers the big question, "How the hell did we get to this point?"'

– **Amanda Thebe**, fitness expert, speaker and author of *Menopocalypse: How I Learned to Thrive During Menopause and How You Can Too*

'Absolutely brilliant! This book makes you stop and think about where we are now, as women; where we have been, and how far we have to go.'

– **Dr Carys Sonnenberg**, GP, BMS-accredited menopause specialist, educator, speaker and author

'*MenoWars* is a much-needed, no-nonsense takedown of the confusion surrounding menopause – finally giving women the science, clarity, and validation we deserve.'

– **Dr Mary Claire Haver**, MD, FACOG, CMP

'*MenoWars* is the book I wish every woman would read. It's an insightful, wide-ranging look at menopause through the ages, across cultures and into the heart of today's medical, political and social conversations. With clarity, warmth and a welcome dose of humour, Fiona separates myth from fact, empowering readers to make informed choices. It's informative without being overwhelming – a smart, essential guide (and a surprisingly entertaining read) for anyone navigating the menopause journey.'

– **Libby Stevenson**, therapeutic wellbeing and
yoga instructor

'The history of women's healthcare is tainted by misogyny, lack of research and the notion that women should just "put up with it", and menopause care is no exception. This brilliant book will guide you like the north star through the modern maze of the menopause world. It explains with clear, no-nonsense language and journalistic meticulousness how we got here; and it gives you the research and the numbers, separating fact from fiction, so that you can make an informed decision when it comes to choosing the right path for your own menopause journey.'

– **Dr Mandy Leonhardt**, GP and BMS-accredited
menopause specialist, and author

'In a time when too many women still face stigma, dismissal or outright neglect, *MenoWars* stands as a rallying cry for change and a lifeline for millions of women who have felt dismissed, confused or unheard. It empowers women not only to advocate for themselves, but to demand better from the systems meant to serve them. This book will leave readers better equipped, better informed, and most importantly, reassured that they are not alone.'

– **Michelle Griffin**, gynaecologist, BBC Health columnist and
founder of MFG Health

'Fiona Clark has written a fabulous book which can only be described as "the menopause book that we have all been waiting for, but didn't know that we were". It's an A to Z on the menopause and a significant contribution to understanding it within the context of history, misogyny, capitalism and politics. I now understand why people think that menopausal women ought to "put up and shut up", but the difference is that Fiona also gives us the tools and language to fight back.'

– **Jane Chelliah**, MBE

'In a sea of menopause advice, *MenoWars* leaves no stone unturned. Sharp, fearless and utterly necessary, Fiona dismantles the misinformation plaguing menopause and gives the reader a solid foundation of knowledge to take away, and she does it with precision and wit. This is not just another menopause book, it's the one that should have come first.'

– **Lou and Jinty**, Womenkind Collective

'The menopause landscape has become commercialised, commodified, competitive and combative. This brilliant, timely book will help you to understand why that has happened, and how to successfully navigate that landscape.'

– **Diane Danzebrink**, menopause advocate and
author of *Making Menopause Matter*

'At times horrifying (leeches on vulvas?), *MenoWars* is exhaustively researched, engagingly written, and most of all, empowering. Fiona Clark makes sense of conflicting evidence and expert opinions, and brings to light the political, marketing and vested interests that influence women's health in ways most of us never realise.'

– **Lynnette Hoffman**, Managing Editor, 'Healthed Australia'

'I loved this book! As "the *Newsnight* anchor of the menopause world", Fiona is perfectly placed to comment on the explosion of information and the deep confusion in the medical world about how to react to the rise of the influencer. A must-read, this is exactly what has been missing – clear, illuminating, researched information, with lived experience adding to an informative and practical resource.

– **Dinah Siman**, author and Menopause Pilates expert

'*MenoWars* is smart, sharp and unafraid to say what so many of us have felt for some time. Honest, necessary and long overdue.'

– **Kate Oakley**, Your Future Fit

'This book is needed! It's written in a hilarious and digestible tone, heavily researched and separating fact from fiction. It's a bold, witty, inclusive and honest piece that everyone must read – after all, everyone will be affected by menopause either directly or indirectly.'

– **Dr Aziza Sesay**, GP educator, Honorary Senior Clinical lecturer,
host, speaker and health content creator

'There is so much going on that is right at this moment – a modern menopause movement is mobilizing around much-needed reforms. Clark brings a critical journalistic lens and unpacks the policies needed to get us back on track. As a US-based advocate, I watch the global menopause landscape carefully; Clark's keen assessments are essential collateral.'

– **Jennifer Weiss-Wolf**, attorney, author and
menstrual health advocate, New York

'Fiona Clark has written what must become the go-to book about menopause, not just for the women themselves going through it, but for doctors, policymakers and even for health journalists like me. From medical misogyny to TikTok misinformation, from health scares about HRT to dementia risks, she looks at the facts, provides the evidence or tells you when it isn't there. She quite simply cuts through the noise and tells you, "it is your menopause, your health, your future, your choices."'

– **Victoria Mcdonald**, Channel 4 Health Correspondent

'A bold, brilliant and necessary book. Fiona unpacks the politics of menopause with journalistic rigour and clarity – challenging the status quo, exposing the gender health gap and empowering women to advocate for better health and a fairer system. This is not your average menopause book – and that's exactly why it matters.'

– **Lavina Mehta MBE**, founder of Feel Good with Lavina, personal trainer, bestselling author, speaker and health campaigner

'Thank you, Fiona, for such an enlightening book that's full of vital and relevant information delivered wit and humour. I absolutely loved it. Now, please, let's get the research we need done! (And, if nothing else, I'm pleased your husband now knows the difference between a Volvo and a vulva!)'

– **Cathy Proctor**, menopause advocate

'The current mantra that "menopause is having a moment" is less about a sudden collective interest in menopause, and more about the economics of selling lotions, potions and promises of longevity. *MenoWars* is an accurate, highly readable look about how we got here and more importantly, a guide to help women navigate information, from misinformation and disinformation. *MenoWars* is a must-read – ideally before the first hot flash hits.'

– **Lauren Streicher MD**, Professor and ObGyn, Northwestern University, author of *Hot Flash Hell*

'In a landscape muddled by misinformation and commercial interests, 'MenoWars' expertly sifts through the noise to deliver clear, no-nonsense insights on menopause that every woman needs. Fiona's engaging writing made it impossible to put down!'

– **Dr Elise Dallas**, GP

'Most women would find it immensely helpful to have a reliable friend to help navigate menopause. They found one in Fiona Clark. She cuts thorough the confusing and conflicting advice in the public arena to give women a balanced, informed, and highly entertaining perspective of what we all should know about menopause.'

– **Pauline M. Maki**, PHD, Professor of Psychiatry, Psychology and Obstetrics & Gynecology, Treasurer International Menopause Society

MenoWars

Money, Misogyny and Mixed Messages

FIONA CLARK

sheldon PRESS

First published by Sheldon Press in 2025
An imprint of John Murray Press

1

This book is for information or educational purposes only and is not intended to act as a substitute for medical advice or treatment. Any person with a condition requiring medical attention should consult a qualified medical practitioner or suitable therapist.

A CIP catalogue record for this title is available from the British Library

Hardback ISBN 978 1 399 82734 8
Trade Paperback ISBN 978 1 399 83096 6
ebook ISBN 978 1 399 82735 5

Typeset by KnowledgeWorks Global Ltd.

Printed and bound in Great Britain by Clays Ltd, Elcograf S.p.A.

John Murray Press policy is to use papers that are natural, renewable and recyclable products and made from wood grown in sustainable forests. The logging and manufacturing processes are expected to conform to the environmental regulations of the country of origin.

John Murray Press
Carmelite House
50 Victoria Embankment
London EC4Y 0DZ

Sheldon Press
Hachette Book Group
123 South Broad Street
Ste 2750
Philadelphia, PA 19109, USA

www.sheldonpress.co.uk

John Murray Press, part of Hodder & Stoughton Limited
An Hachette UK company

The authorised representative in the EEA is Hachette Ireland, 8 Castlecourt Centre, Dublin 15, D15 XTP3, Ireland (email: info@hbgi.ie)

To my husband, son, daughter-in-law, who have patiently borne the embarrassment and indignity of me talking endlessly and publicly about vaginas – my own and in general – and have emerged relatively unscathed. I take it as a small but significant victory that my husband now knows the difference between a Volvo and a vulva. That's a win!

Hell hath no fury like a menopausal woman.

– said Shakespeare never (and he really didn't
but he should have!)

Contents

Foreword by Dr Naomi Potter

Way back in early 2020, I sat down in front of my phone to do my first ever Instagram live chat with Fiona on menopause and hormone replacement therapy. It was early days for these sorts of things and she was among the first to be doing in-depth but accessible interviews with healthcare experts about menopause. I was a bit nervous, but we made it through, and a grand total of 47 people watched it live. How things have changed!

Social media platforms, and the number of voices on them, has grown exponentially as has the number of opinions and views expressed – which can sometimes make it difficult for women to tell the fact from the fiction.

Who better to sort the way through the maze than Fiona. She has a science background and spent the first 20 years or so of her career as a news and current affairs reporter, producer and supervising producer for the Australian Broadcasting Corporation (ABC). She was a reporter in the Soviet Union covering the August 1991 coup and then returned to Sydney to work on the ABC's equivalent of *Newsnight*, where she covered a range of topics from health to domestic and international politics. She left the ABC in 2001 and moved to medical publishing – just before the controversial WHI study landed in 2002. Since then she has held various positions including section editor and editor-in-chief and has written for prestigious journals including *The Lancet*.

And for the past seven or so years though she has dedicated herself to menopause and has done around 1,000 interviews on the topic with experts from across the globe, earning herself the moniker of 'the *Newsnight* of menopause'. She has also set up a charity called the Menopause Research and Education Fund (MREF) with the mission of supporting research and delivering education to medical professionals and consumers alike. So, suffice to say she has had a bird's eye view of the menopause landscape as its unfolded over the past few years and in this book she's taken a step back to examine where we are now and the ramifications.

It is indeed a book that captures the zeitgeist. But it's not just about how we came to this point in time with so many voices. Using her years of investigative reporting skills she's taken on some quite heavy topics. With more than 200 reports and references gone through and some 30 plus interviews conducted she's looked at how menopause impacts on women's earning capacity, ability to stay in work and our productivity and the cost to the economy.

She has looked at how we are now the target of marketers and the growth of the Femtech sector and the possible implications for data protection and our privacy, and how we can overcome some of these issues in the future. She has also tapped into thorny issues like gendered ageism and the importance of declaring conflicts of interest when it comes to policymaking.

And she's also looked at the enduring misogyny in medicine when it comes to women's reproductive health as well as the paucity of funding for women's health research and the lack of women in research trials that persists today, all of which have contributed to gender data gaps and a shorter 'health span' that sees us living almost a decade longer in poor health than men.

Some of the things that affect our health in the last decades of life are tackled in the third section of the book, when Fiona turns to address the silent changes that happen around menopause that we may not even notice that affect our bones, brain, bladders and vaginas as well as our heart and metabolic risk. She looks at the current debates on how to handle these, bust some myths, and then delivers the practical expert advice from those in the know on how to improve our own health. These are so important because we know that women are twice as likely to develop dementia later in life than men and we're also far more likely to experience a fragility fracture as a result of osteoporosis, become incontinent and, although we usually associate heart attacks with men, it is among the leading causes of death for women. So, if we want to keep ourselves as fit and healthy as we can, for as long as we can, this section is a must read.

The last section looks at how we can find common ground and advocate for better health systems and also for ourselves. This is vital as many of the women I see still don't know enough about menopause and, even if they do, they are still confused about what their options are. And sadly, they often feel guilty or ashamed for seeking help for their symptoms. And one of the main messages from the opening paragraph of this book to the very last is that this is your body, your choice, and no one else's opinion matters. It is between you and your doctor.

Unfortunately, we are far from having perfect health systems, even in the richest of countries, so it's time to start thinking about how we right the historical wrongs, fill the data gaps and get better services, access and treatments for all women because menopause affects every person born with ovaries at some stage of their life, as well as the people who care for them. This book is an important marker in focusing on what matters now and how we can make things better for in the future.

Fiona has a taken some very difficult topics but combined them with her personal experience where relevant and those of others to make them approachable, and she's done it with wit and levity. I'm so pleased to have shared part of my journey with her and can't think of a better, objective person to have tackled so many aspects of such an enormous topic. It'll make you angry, it'll make you laugh and hopefully it'll inspire you to a better future health.

Dr Naomi Potter
BMS Accredited Menopause Specialist
BSc MSc MBBS DRCOG DFSRH MRCGP BMS
Founder/Clinical Director, Menopause Care Ltd
Co-author of the 2023 Book of the Year prize-winner Menopausing

Foreword by Dr Vikram Talaulikar

I first met Fiona about nine years ago when we were discussing clinical services for post-reproductive healthcare at a roundtable. It struck me that, although Fiona was invited to the meeting as a stakeholder, she was genuinely passionate about transforming the landscape of menopause care and bringing about a real culture 'change' in how everyone viewed the 'menopause transition' so that individuals allround the country could benefit from such a change. This book is one among the many milestones in that journey for change.

Fiona starts the book by describing what we know about the menopause transition at present. In the first three chapters, she takes us through the physiology behind the changes individuals experience, the symptomatology and how clinicians or scientists diagnose the various phases of the transition. She describes the magnitude of challenges we face in relation to menopause care of the future.

With life expectancy for women on the rise, most women will experience menopause transition and will spend a significant number of years of their life in the postmenopausal phase. The second part of the book delves into societal and political implications of post-reproductive health during menopause. It addresses issues such as misogyny and underrepresentation when it comes to menopause research and funding. Over the past 10–15 years, there has been a significant increase in conversations and information exchange about menopause and HRT in the Western world. This has been brought about by healthcare professionals and organisations, but also by health campaigners, celebrities and social media influencers in the menopause space. Most of this has been positive. But there are also some negatives. Not all information in the public domain is accurate and facts can be blurred or presented in a way by individuals to suit an agenda. Robust scientific evidence related to menopause treatments can be scarce in certain clinical situations and cherry picking of favourable studies and presenting personal opinions as scientific facts can misguide individuals/consumers regarding the best interventions for them (with the potential to lead to clinical harm).

Businesses around the world have sensed the opportunity in the menopause market and there seems to be a far greater rush to produce, advertise or recommend solutions, supplements and new technological innovations for problems related to the menopause even before we have enough scientific evidence for some of what actually happens during the transition! Fiona covers the commercialisation of menopause in her next chapter and addresses issues related to lack of need for robust evidence of safety/efficacy and regulation in this sector of industry.

In the next section of the book, Fiona focuses on long-term health impact of menopause on various organ systems of the body – brain, heart, blood vessels, bones, muscles, skin, metabolism and genitourinary system. There are several lifestyle and/or medical interventions which can be considered as options to improve long-term health and prevent negative impact of premature, early or natural age menopause. Knowledge is key when making the right choices!

The final section of the book explores what can be done to make this phase of life better for individuals especially those who face ethnic, financial, socio-cultural or geographical barriers to good quality healthcare and health education. It is important that the momentum that has been gained with people advocating for themselves in the menopause space is not lost and that campaigners continue to demand better policies and changes to health systems from policymakers and politicians to make further progress. With the right help and support – menopause can be the most productive phase in the life of an individual where they can pass on their experience and knowledge to make a positive contribution to society.

Many people are concerned about certain issues that affect them, but few have the strength and courage to take concrete action to try and resolve them. Fiona certainly was not going to sit and wait for others to act when it came to educating healthcare professionals about menopause and fund raising for more menopause research! That was how the Menopause Research and Education Fund charity was born. Thanks to the efforts of Fiona and Diane Danzebrink (a prolific menopause campaigner herself), we founded the charity in 2024 and it has already educated more than 1,000 professionals across the world in menopause care.

There is still a long way to go before we make good quality, evidence-based, easily accessible menopause care available to everyone without any barriers, but until that happens, I am sure Fiona will be right at the forefront campaigning for better! As she says in her book – we all need to strive for the change together!

Dr Vikram Talaulikar
MD, FRCOG, PhD
Associate Specialist, Reproductive Medicine Unit, UCLH
Hon. Associate Professor in Women's Health at UCL
Trainer for BMS and FSRH menopause modules

Preface

Back in 2020, on a chilly October afternoon, menopause activist Kate Duffy, her two daughters and I met up under the watchful gaze of a statue of Dame Millicent Fawcett, suffragette and social campaigner, outside the Houses of Parliament in Westminster. Armed with a loud-hailer and sporting our Menopause Support 'Make Menopause Matter' T-shirts, we yelled that slogan at those passing by and had a good laugh while doing so.

What a difference a year makes. Just 365 days later, the scene in Parliament Square was very, very different. Hundreds of women turned up to call for better awareness of menopause and a better deal for menopausal women. There were MPs, doctors, celebrities and grassroots campaigners, all championing the cause in spirit of unity and sisterly love. Menopause was indeed 'having a moment'. It made the evening news and front pages of the daily papers. Menopause had come of age. But what had changed to get to this point and where have we ended up since then?

It's very easy to say it's the 'Davina effect'. The celebrity TV pre-senter's first Channel 4 documentary on menopause had come out in May 2021, and was a rallying call for many. But this didn't happen in just five months. The path to Parliament Square has a long history that's been built on the hard work of many over the years whose lives have, in one way or another, been affected by 'the menopause'.

Since then the information landscape, if you will, has changed. Social media and the rise of influencers, medical or otherwise, has metaphori-cally thrown a hand grenade into the ivory tower of the medical estab-lishment, leaving it to play catch-up when it comes to controlling the narrative and the delivery of evidence-based menopause information. (Now, before you get angry about the use of the term 'influencer' – I too hate it, and after 40 years as a journalist, I find it offensive to be called one myself – but that is the commonly used term, so let's not take it as an insult but simply for what it is: part of the current vernacular.)

While there are many positives to this new democratisation of medical information, it also has its downside. When different parties, some with huge followings, send conflicting messages, it creates a sea of confusion that leaves both doctors and the public struggling to know who the 'trusted' voice is.

The UK has also seen a parade of menopause ambassadors, HRT tsars, parliamentary reports and recommendations that are paving the way for a better, healthier future for all those born with ovaries who, if they live long enough, will go through menopause. And there have been some concrete changes too – like the introduction of the HRT prepayment certificate in England that's made Menopause Hormone Therapies cheaper for all those who need it.

And it's not just here. Across the pond in the US there were significant pledges of cash from the Biden administration for research and a push is now on, perhaps optimistically given the Trump administration's dislike for what it sees as 'gendered wokism', for legislative changes that will protect the rights of menopausal women and ensure there is no discrimination against them.

In Australia, my birth nation, there's recently been a Senate inquiry looking into menopause that has made some substantial recommendations, many of which were accepted by the government and could improve access to information and treatments for women down under.

But we still have a very long way to go.

There are socio-economic, ethnic and cultural disparities that need to be addressed across the globe. It's expected that by 2030 there will be approximately 1.2 billion women around the world in menopause,[1] and many countries don't have the access to information or treatments anywhere near what we have in Western countries.

Menopause has an effect not just on our quality of life and relationships but also on our economy and democracy. I say that in the sense of equity and the ability to take part in society in a fully functional manner – in good health and able to work without the fear of prejudice and discrimination.

And, it affects our health. Not only can the symptoms that hit us in perimenopause be debilitating for some, with depression, vasomotor symptoms, and joint and muscle pain wreaking havoc on their lives, it also heralds a series of silent changes that impact our future health. Our bones can become weaker, putting us at risk of breaking a hip or fracturing a spine. Our bladders leak, and incontinence is up there in the top three reasons women are admitted to care facilities. Our risk of metabolic diseases rises as we no longer handle blood sugar as we as we did in the past, and there are changes to our cholesterol, triglycerides and blood pressure that put us at great risk of a heart attack or stroke. We know that by the age of 65 a woman's risk of a heart attack is equal to a man's, yet we are still less likely to have the symptoms recognised or be treated for it, and are more likely to die as a result.

And then there's brain health. We are at greater risk of dementia and it's not just because we're living longer.

All of these factors combine to see women spend 25 per cent more time in ill health than our male counterparts. That equates to nearly a decade more of our lives spent in poor health.

This is why menopause is important. It affects every aspect of life for every person born female who lives long enough, and all those who care for them. But, the amount of money spent on menopause research is virtually nil in the grand scheme of things. Women's health in general attracts around 10 per cent of publicly allocated research funding and the majority of that is spent on breast and reproductive cancers. In the US in 2020, only 5 per cent of global research and development (R&D) funding was allocated to women's health research, according to a study in *Nature*.[2] The authors said 4 per cent of this was spent on women's cancers and 1 per cent went on 'all other women-specific health conditions, with 25% of that further limited to fertility research'. US-based brain researcher Lisa Mosconi has said it's impossible to tell what goes on menopause, but in the UK an analysis on funding allocated by the National Institute for Health and Care Research (NIRH) shows that between 1993 and September 2024 there were 8,919 studies funded and just 33 of them mentioned the word 'menopause'. That equates to 0.37 per cent of the studies and attracted just 0.29 per cent of the £6,23 billion or so allocated in funding.[3] This is one of the main reasons activist Diane Danzebrink, reproductive health specialist Vikram Talaulikar and I started the Menopause Research and Education Fund in 2023 – we have too many unanswered questions on menopause health and not enough resources allocated to them to get them answered. This needs to change.

Attitudes to menopause need to change too. Like the abortion debate, everyone has an opinion on what women should or shouldn't be doing with our bodies when it comes to hormone therapy. There are claims that menopause has become 'over-medicalised' and arguments that taking hormones is a cop-out; after all, women have gone through it since day dot, so what's wrong with us? The 'suck it up, princess' argument.

But all this 'sucking it up' and lack of research has fuelled a massive and rapidly growing market for supplements, self-help courses and unregulated devices as well as multiple new professions including menopause coaches, doulas and workplace policy advisors. It's an environment that is poorly regulated in terms of standards or safety. This too needs to change.

These are just some of the topics this book looks at as it documents the evolving menopause landscape. I've been fortunate to have spoken to some of the key players who have helped shaped 'the change' (pun intended!) so far, looking at the challenges we're facing, what's been achieved and what's still on the 'to-do' list, and it's long. The aim of this book is to help you navigate your way through what can be a complicated maze so you can do your menopause your way, while ensuring your future health.

Terminology

Throughout the book I have used the term 'women'. I know it's not ideal for all, but I am using it inclusively, as shorthand for all those born with ovaries and those who identify as women, non-binary or gender non-conforming.

I have also opted to use the term Menopause Hormone Therapy (MHT) or simply hormone therapy (HT) for what is known as Hormone Replacement Therapy (HRT) in the UK, unless in a direct quote, as these are now the accepted terms in most parts of the world.

The other term that differs between continents is hot flushes or hot flashes. This time I'm going with the UK unless it's a direct quote – so hot flushes it is! And unless otherwise stated, all dollar references ($) are US dollars.

Read on, and I hope you enjoy it.

Introduction

You may have found yourself wondering what on earth is going on in the world of menopause. What was once a nice, supportive space that you'd think everybody would agree on has quickly descended into what looks like a war of words, with experts battling it out in the media and on social media. This book looks at how we came to this point. How the rise of the 'influencer' (and yes, I hate that word too) has thrown a grenade into the ivory tower of the medical establishment, leaving it blinking like a deer in the headlights of a fast approaching bullet train. It says claims have been made that are not backed by evidence, and those who have made them claim the establishment is out of date, out of touch and have acted like gatekeepers on information for the benefit of their own members while women have been left floundering and desperately looking for answers to the symptoms they've been suffering with. They say they were filling a void in a system that was failing women.

This book aims to look at how this has happened, the effects it has had on trust, why it's important economically, socially and culturally, and in terms of your long-term health. And, importantly, how you can navigate your way through it to ensure that the many decades (it could be literally 50 years or more) you spend as postmenopausal women will be as healthy and productive as they can be.

It is not a book that is looking at who is right or wrong – it is stepping back and looking at the landscape, the barriers, the implications, and posing ways that we can bridge the divide and come back to a centre point where we can all work together with common goals to improve women's health.

Ultimately though, it is about you. Women have forever been the focus of everyone's opinions from cradle to grave. How you can free yourself from everyone else's opinions about menopause and make sure you have a good menopause – your body, your choices, your way.

The book is in four parts. The first part looks at how we came to be where we are. The second part looks at the politics, culture and misogyny and why menopause matters economically as well as the rise of the menomarket, health and data gaps and the question of trust, disclosure and conflicts of interest. The third part moves on to why menopause is important to your health – the silent changes that can affect your heart, brain, metabolic health and genitourinary health (vaginas and bladders) and what you can do to help yourself. And finally, the fourth part looks at politics and power and where we can find common ground. It explores how you can advocate for change for yourself in a health system that still has a long way to go in terms of education on menopause and listening to women's voices.

This is for you and the generations to come. It's not just a menopause moment, it's a movement – a revolution if you like – and you are at its centre.

1

WHAT THE HELL IS GOING ON?

There are as many opinions as there are experts.

– Franklin D. Roosevelt

1

Ovaries, opinions and the rise of the 'influencer'

'I'll rip your ovaries out and feed them to the nearest cat!' The first time I heard this phrase as a teenager it was delivered from the lips of my godmother. I don't remember what I'd done to deserve such a threat, but it literally made me laugh out loud. She could have gone for the heart or throat, but the fact that she chose the ovaries shows just how significant those tiny little egg-producing organs, about the size of plum tomatoes, are to our purpose in life – to reproduce. It's how we're defined – our essence. Before menopause our health is called 'reproductive health'. Postmenopause, it's 'post-reproductive health' – a term that makes me cringe every time I read it. I know it makes medical sense because things change with every stage of reproductive life – but it still makes my hackles rise because I'd prefer to not to be categorised by my ability to reproduce. Yet here we are.

And no matter what stage of our reproductive life we're at, everyone has an opinion on it. What menstrual products you should use, when you should be allowed to have sex, who you should have sex with, if you should be married when you have sex, if you should take the pill or use a 'natural' form of contraception, when you should get pregnant, how many kids you should or shouldn't have, and how you should deliver them. If you have an epidural or a caesarean – well, God help you, you took 'the easy way out' (I had a caesarean, by the way – it probably saved both our lives). And then there are abortions: should or shouldn't you be allowed to terminate your pregnancy and, if so, how and when? And at the other end of the reproductive spectrum, when you're really thinking 'enough already, surely by now it's my body, my choice?' we get arguments about taking Hormone Replacement Therapy (HRT) as they call it in the UK, or Menopause Hormone Therapy (MHT), as they call it elsewhere. If you do decide to take it you get slammed for not being tough enough 'to ride it out', after all, 'it's natural' and every woman's been through it since we crawled out of the primordial slime, so what's wrong with you? Then come the arguments about whether you're too young to take it, or too old, not to mention 'it'll give you cancer'. But if you don't take it you're doomed to spend your dotage in a wheelchair with a broken hip, incontinence and dementia – that is, of course, if you don't die of a heart attack first. Even at menopause, women's bodies and what we do with them are everyone's business but our own, and it seems everyone is talking about them.

We live in the era of the social media influencer – medical or otherwise. It is the nomenclature *du jour*, even though it may appear derogatory when applied to experts in their field. Despite the term, they are there, en masse, experts or otherwise, across the globe sharing their stories, opinions or information on every available platform online. Some are selling their 'clinically proven', menopause 'tick'-approved products that claim to help us through every facet of this transition from hair loss and itchy, sagging skin to hot flushes, weight loss and anxiety. Others are sharing their personal wisdom, providing coaching, counselling or workplace support, and others are educating women on what their lifestyle or medical options are. Some are medically qualified and have hundreds of thousands, even millions, of followers who, after years of feeling isolated, lost and like they're quietly losing their marbles, are now relieved to find that they're not alone – there are other people out there who understand them, or are going through exactly what they're going through, and there are options that can help them.

And there's been a tsunami of information made available on multiple platforms. In the UK alone since 2018 there have been about half a dozen TV documentaries, the most famous being the ones featuring British TV celebrity Davina McCall. These are credited with creating what's known as the 'Davina effect' which is said to have given rise to a 42 per cent jump in the number of prescriptions issued for menopause hormone therapy (MHT) in the year after it went to air.[1] In the US there's been a good handful too, culminating in 2024 with *The M Factor* which features a range of high-profile women's health advocates, researchers and healthcare practitioners discussing the effects menopause has had on them or their patients, and the options available to help.

Baffling bits of science that were once the exclusive fodder of the medical establishment have been explained and discussed in one-minute social media reels. Facebook groups are filled with tens of thousands of women asking questions, podcasts have been launched, YouTube channels created, Threads and Substacks written, along with numerous books – some by menopause advocates, some by doctors, some by celebrities, and some by a mix of all three. And barely a week goes by without an article in a newspaper or magazine, or someone on the radio or TV talking about some aspect of menopause. In fact, there's so much out there that one PR guru told me it was becoming increasingly difficult for him to get a menopause story placed because the editors thought it was *passé* and a saturated market. Newspapers may well be sick of running stories on it, but what can't be denied is that this past decade or so has seen some remarkable changes in the menopause landscape and the way it's viewed culturally, economically and politically.

Veteran campaigner Diane Danzebrink, who started Menopause Support and the Make Menopause Matter campaign, says 'there is definitely more awareness of the word "menopause". There is certainly a lot more conversation, particularly on social media. When I started my research back in 2013, I was researching online forums. There wasn't TikTok and Instagram, but of course, now social media is so much a part of so many people's lives. There's a lot more information out there and we have definitely seen more people raising their voices in terms of campaigning.'

It didn't take long for others like Katie Taylor (The Latte Lounge), Kate Duffy (Meno Mave), Jane Anne James (@janemhdg) and Elizabeth Carr-Ellis (Pausitivity) to join the space. And over time what started as grassroots campaigns around the kitchen tables of a handful of people across the UK, many of whom were driven by their own less than ideal personal experiences and a desire for no one to go through what they went through, grew quickly and by the early 2020s it had hit its stride. Celebrities, doctors, politicians, journalists and broadcasters joined forces on World Menopause Day in 2021 and again in 2022 to rally outside Parliament House in London to lobby the government for change. Sporting T-shirts with 'Make Menopause Matter' and carrying signs saying 'Join the Menopause Revolution', their unified chorus hit the front pages of national newspapers, spawning government reviews and numerous reports, as well as the appointment of a menopause tsar and women's health and women's workplace ambassadors (see Chapter 11).

Labour Member of Parliament Carolyn Harris, who has been at the forefront of pushing for changes for menopausal women in Westminster, described the 2021 rally as 'a momentous day. As we gathered in Parliament Square, there were cheers of joy and tears of relief; . . . you could feel the utter delight in the atmosphere as women celebrated what they perceived as a victory.'[2]

And it soon spread its wings, helping to fuel menopause conversations in the US, Canada, New Zealand and Australia. In the US, political heavyweights like Maria Schriver (a member of the powerful Kennedy family and former first lady of California) joined forces with the former first lady Jill Biden and leading menopause researchers, doctors and health advocates to successfully push for a commitment on funding for much-needed menopause research. They were joined by celebrities like Halle Berry who shouted loudly on Capitol Hill 'I'm in menopause and it's OK'. Another former first lady, Michelle Obama started speaking out about her experience, as did Oprah, Drew Barrymore, Naomi Watts, and a host of others. And down under, the Australian Senate held a public inquiry to help determine what direction the country should take to better support menopausal women, which resulted in the funding of a public health campaign.[3]

Menopause wasn't just 'having a moment' as the headlines had cried,[4] it was way past that. 'I feel like whatever was making this "a moment" is now cementing it into a movement,' says Jennifer Weiss-Wolf, a US-based lawyer, menopause advocate and author. This isn't the first time in the past 50 years or so that menopause and its first-line treatment – hormone therapy – has been on the agenda, though. In the '70s it was big for what we'd now consider to be all the wrong reasons – the elixir of youth – a way to avoid the 'inevitable decay' and becoming a 'castrate', as Robert Wilson wrote in his book *Feminine Forever* (see Chapter 6). It had another moment in the late 1990s/early 2000s when actor Lauren Hutton was extolling its virtues for a similar reason. *Newsweek* ran an article entitled 'Why is Lauren Hutton smiling? Hormones!'. They called her 'a paid hormone spokeswoman' and quoted her as saying, 'I can usually pick out the women who are taking it because they look much younger than their age, and they don't look . . . shrunk or dried up.'[5] (I guess the payments helped her smile a bit too!)

But this time it's different, says Weiss-Wolf, who has worked successfully to get various US states to lift the luxury or 'pink tax' on tampons and is now turning her considerable brain to menopause policy. 'There's a generational drum beat to it' that, she says, is being fuelled by the attacks on women's reproductive rights in the US, the dearth of research on women's health and menopause in particular, and the lack of educated medical professionals and education for women on menopause. 'We need new policy momentum to right some of these wrongs . . . So, what's different this time is something about the generational call that feels very powerful, and because it's in the context of a lot of other women's health issues that are under fire, it seems less likely to go away.'

And as great as this movement and the democratisation of information that's come with it is, it has sent shock waves through the medical establishment who have literally not known how or where to respond to what they see are 'off piste' claims that are being made about hormone therapies. Members of menopause societies across the globe are increasingly worried that some of the messages being sent to women are being oversold, outstrip the current evidence base or are scaremongering, over-playing the risks in order to sell other 'alternative' or 'hormone-free' products. Key among their concerns are commonly cited views that have entered the mainstream including that menopause should be regarded as a hormone deficiency that needs to be treated, and that menopause hormone therapy will prevent conditions like type 2 diabetes, dementia and heart disease – or on the other end of the scale, that MHT will cause cancer, so should be avoided like the plague.

'We're in a bit of a pickle,' says chair of the British Menopause Society (BMS), consultant gynaecologist Janice Rymer, who has been working in women's health and prescribing hormone therapy since the 1990s. 'Everybody's saying every symptom between the age of 40 to the 60s is due to the ovarian failure therefore you need oestrogen – which is wrong. And then the other thing is, everybody needs testosterone. And again, wrong. So, those are the two biggest challenges at the moment. Now, I think HRT is wonderful, don't get me wrong. I've been in the HRT world for a very long time and I think it's great and it makes such a difference to so many women, but it's the expectations that are being set that are the problem. Now, everybody says "take HRT and you're going to go back to your 20-year-old self," and so poor women are having these expectations that everything's going to be solved by that, when it's not always the case.'

Even though they're concerned, they've found it difficult to respond and weren't even sure if it was their responsibility. But after a long period of watching quietly from the sidelines, various menopause societies have started to raise their voices to question the narratives even if it is mostly within their own 'ivory towers'. Since 2022, the BMS and more recently the International Menopause Society (IMS) have issued position statements and white papers for their members aimed at countering claims that MHT prevents dementia[6] and heart disease,[7] that all women should be on testosterone,[8] and clarifying issues on dosing levels.[9] The IMS thought addressing the current controversies was so important that it made it the central focus of its 2024 international conference in Melbourne and issued a white paper for World Menopause Day to coincide with it.[10] The introduction sums up the situation we find ourselves in: 'After many years of neglect, we have finally seen long overdue unprecedented attention given to menopause in the popular media, empowering women to seek care for menopause symptoms. Yet the media and even academic literature present polarised views on its management. These contrasting views often leave women feeling confused and disempowered rather than supported through their menopause transition and susceptible to unproven marketed products.'

The authors go on to say: 'Very few therapeutic medical interventions have generated as much controversy, and very few have waxed and waned in popularity as much as MHT . . . Opinions about MHT appear to be driven as much by the sociocultural climate as they are by the emerging evidence from clinical trials' and 'the widespread dissemination of misinformation and disinformation may encourage some of these women to request MH [Menopause Hormones] from their HPs [healthcare professionals] purely to maintain skin, nail and hair quality and/or for potential primary prevention benefits such as cardiovascular and brain health, for which there is not currently an indication. This has been one of the key issues which has caused recent controversy given that MH is not currently recommended solely for primary prevention.'

While it's admirable that they've taken these steps, most doctors aren't members of these organisations, which means these groups are largely, unfortunately, talking among themselves. Just to put that into perspective, as of December 2024 there were 54,000 GPs in the UK and 7,133 obstetricians and gynaecologists, but in January 2025 the BMS had just 2,500 members.[11] In the US the Menopause Society has 7,900 members but there are 527,168 primary healthcare physicians[12] and of those around 118,000 are family care physicians[13] and 20,000 are gynaecologists.[14] Suffice to say, it's not a huge reach in either country.

When it comes to informing the public about menopause, that's beyond their remit, Rymer says: 'We are a society for healthcare professionals, and I think we've just got to do what we do and do it well. And we don't want to blow it.' She explains that their responses to their members take time because they must, quite rightly, be measured and accurate, and the doctors involved are unpaid volunteers who do this in what little spare time they have after work. Unfortunately though those time lapses leave ample space for claims to take root and flourish and, to mix my metaphors, once a horse has bolted it's very hard to catch, let alone put back in the stable.

But it's not just the public who are getting their information from social media – doctors are too. How do I know? Because when I do my interviews with experts, many of the audience are doctors and they often ask questions. So, if they're getting the same messages as the public and reinforcing them to their patients, the divisions will only get wider and a failure to engage is unlikely to help.

Danzebrink thinks 'they've been left in the wake of the rise of social media. I don't think that they grasped the importance of it anywhere near quickly enough. They've not used it to their advantage and that is a huge missed opportunity. They have not made themselves the trusted voices in this space, and ultimately, they've been left in the wake of influencers . . . And if you're behind the curve, well, basically you are in the dust.'

This is especially important because many doctors have very little education on menopause – just like the rest of us.

This can't go on though, gynaecologist turned Femtech guru Michelle Griffin says: 'Society is moving at a pace that our systems don't keep up with so we can't just sit there in the ivory tower and keep saying, "well, medicine doesn't work like that, we can't respond to you." No, it can't work like that, we have to change the system, the culture, and have more flexibility in the medical knowledge being offered so that we can adapt more readily to the pace of change and what's happening.'

One debate that did make it smack bang onto the feminist agenda in *Ms.* magazine in the US was the response to a four-part series of articles on menopause in the medical journal *The Lancet*.[15] One paper in the series stood out and drew the ire of a swathe of medical professionals from across the globe, and this is why.

First up there was an article that accompanied the series that explained the paper's lead author, Australian obstetrician and gynaecologist Professor Martha Hickey, was taking a 'feminist perspective on menopause, which includes normalising this life transition and challenging the prevalent idea that it marks a period of physical and mental decline'.[16]

Then came an editorial called 'Time for a balanced conversation about menopause'[17] which, perhaps ironically, *The Lancet* said was part of a 'redoubling' of its effort to redress the historic poor treatment of women in research including reversing 'the longstanding gender biases in medicine'. It went on to say 'over-medicalisation of menopause and promotion of MHT as a panacea is unhelpful and only serves to divide opinions further. It is time for a sensible conversation about menopause to enable informed, individualised decision making on optimal management of this transition.'

Next came the paper itself, called 'An empowerment model for managing the menopause', which said: 'Rather than focusing on menopause as an endocrine deficiency, we propose an empowerment model that recognises factors modifying the experience, in which the patient is an expert in their own condition and the healthcare worker supports the patient to become an equal and active partner in managing their own care.' Sounds great, you'd think, but then the authors signalled these as key points:[18]

- Most women navigate menopause without the need for medical treatment.
- Over-medicalisation of menopause can lead to disempowerment and over-treatment.
- New tools are available to support the empowerment of women to navigate the menopause transition.
- Empowerment is likely to confer benefits for women across socioeconomic and geographical locations, health services, and economies.

If it were unity and support they were after, it's certainly not what they found. Those first two points were the killers, ruffling feathers across the globe and none more so than those in the US where a strong 'menoposse' of like-minded doctors had formed. They were particularly incensed and their rebuttal took no prisoners.

Leader of the menoposse was Mary Claire Haver MD, a board-certified obstetrician and gynaecologist in Texas who had just written a book on menopause. Haver – who has around 7 million followers on various social media platforms, sees patients and runs a supplement company as well – managed to get hold of an embargoed copy and even though she'd been forewarned, her response was visceral: 'So, I get it, I open it, I'm reading it. I was in the car with my husband, and expletives were flying out of my mouth. I had just written a book on menopause so I knew the data backwards and forwards because the data in it was sound, and I was like, "this is the most cherry-picked piece of work I've ever read in my life." But then as I read through I started crying because I thought this is going to hurt women.

'I was so sad. I just went into a little ball. I couldn't even talk. And I just thought . . . all these doctors who are seeing all this stuff in social media and who don't know what to do, and who don't know how to sift through the data and know what is based on studies done 20 something years ago versus what's current and don't understand, are going to read this and think, "Oh, here we go again," and put them on an antidepressant . . . So, it took me a couple of days and then I got mad, and then I was furious, and then we started a bigger group chat.

We started calling our friends. We waited till it was released so that we could talk about it openly. And then there was this push asking "what can we do?"'

A couple of the members in the group wrote a response and sent it to *The Lancet*, but Haver says they got no reply, in fact they 'wouldn't even acknowledge they'd got it', she says. It was 'a stone wall'. Then they sent it to *The New York Times* who also refused to publish it, saying it wasn't their role to respond to articles in medical journals. Undeterred they moved on and pulled together an article instead, and Jennifer Weiss-Wolf pitched it to feminist icon Gloria Steinem's *Ms.* magazine who gave it the green light. *Ms.* is the magazine she started in the 1970s,[19] and for those of you who are too young to remember who Gloria Steinem is, she is one of the US's foremost feminist thinkers, an author and activist who has fought for women's and children's rights as well as race and gender equity since the late 1960's. At the tender age of 91 (at the time of writing), she is still a consulting editor.

The article had the signatures of more than 250 doctors backing it and they picked four points from *The Lancet* piece to take to task:

1. Most women navigate menopause without the need for medical treatments.

They claimed this was inaccurate, citing statistics that showed 90 per cent of women were never educated about menopause, so they don't even know what they have. Even if they did, 73 per cent don't know they can treat their symptoms and only 7 per cent of medical practitioners in the US felt competent to even treat a menopausal woman.

2. During the menopausal transition, women should 'challenge self-critical beliefs, which can . . . make [hot] flushes worse'.

This, they wrote, was 'tone-deaf' and perpetuated the 'it's all in her head' narrative that has been used for decades to dismiss women who present with physical symptoms in the clinical setting. They added, 'These symptoms result from disruptions in the body's thermoregulatory system and are not psychological in nature.'

Cognitive behavioural therapy (CBT) has been shown to be effective in helping manage hot flushes, according to the Menopause Society's latest 'Non-hormone Therapy Position Statement',[20] but it should not be a panacea or recommended as first-line treatment, the doctors argued. MHT is the gold standard. This is also the recommendation of the 2024 NICE guidelines – offer MHT and consider CBT as an option, especially for those who can't take hormone therapies.[21]

> *3. On the basis of scarce data, we found no compelling evidence that risk of anxiety, bipolar disorder, or psychosis is universally elevated over the menopause transition.*

This quote floored them and they countered saying: 'Research has shown a four-fold increase in risk of depressive symptoms, and a two-and-a-half-fold increase in the diagnosis of major depressive disorder – risks greatest in women with vasomotor symptoms. Also, the rate of antidepressant use for women has been shown to double after age 40.' They saved this for last . . .

> *4. Over-medicalization of menopause can lead to disempowerment and over-treatment.*

This, they said, smacked of medical misogyny and perpetuated the 'suck it up sister' attitude that women should simply suffer through the multiple effects declining levels of oestrogen have on the body.

'There is no debate in medicine whether other processes associated with aging should be offered treatment with modern medical solutions. A notable double standard seems to emerge regarding female aging and menopause,' they wrote. 'The painful reality for many patients is that clinicians repeatedly fail to recognise their symptoms of menopause that extend beyond the classic vasomotor symptom of hot flashes. These include inflammatory conditions, cardiac and neurological issues, sexual dysfunction, and sleep and mood disorders. Women frequently find themselves referred to numerous specialists to address the multitude of symptoms associated with menopause, with each symptom being tackled individually; clinicians unable to connect the dots, akin to playing a game of whack-a-mole with symptoms.' The result? 'A cabinet full of prescription medications, costly medical bills and negligible relief. This is the true over-medicalisation of menopause' – which of course goes back to the first point – they're getting treated for multiple things when menopause could be the issue, but they have no idea it is.

It's a powerful argument, backed up by some interesting facts on prescribing data that show that the percentage of women using MHT is now much lower than it was at the beginning of this century. So, let me take you back in time to 2002 to find out why. That year the Women's Health Initiative (WHI), a huge trial run by the National Institutes of Health (NIH) in the US, released the first round of data from two randomised, placebo-controlled trials of hormone therapy in postmenopausal women. It included 10,739 women who'd had a hysterectomy (removal of their uterus) and 16,608 who still had one. Those without a uterus were on an oestrogen-only arm of the study and the rest were on oestrogen and a progestin (a synthetic form of progesterone, the hormone that protects the lining of the womb from becoming too thick and increasing the risk of endometrial cancer). The hormones they used were a type of oestrogen called 'conjugated equine urine' (CEE) – yes, the old-fashioned one made from pregnant mare's pee; and the progestin was medroxyprogesterone acetate. (A boring detail perhaps, but important!) Those two groups were divided into active treatment (those who were given hormones) and placebo (sugar pill) arms.

After five years of following these women, the trials were abruptly stopped because they found that there was an increased risk of breast cancer, coronary heart disease, stroke and deep vein thrombosis (blood clots) in those taking the hormones. Headlines in newspapers screamed 'HRT increases the risk of breast cancer by 26%' and women across the globe made a universal beeline for the loo and immediately flushed their tablets away en masse. (Spare a thought for the fish!) I remember this well. I'd just left the Australian Broadcasting Corporation and moved into medical publishing and was plunged headfirst into a menopausal mess that I had no idea about, but I remember the differences in coverage between the mainstream and medical press couldn't have been starker with the medical side trying very hard to stop the panic.

The mainstream press reported the percentage increases, which were a 29 per cent increased risk of developing heart disease and a

26 per cent chance of being diagnosed with breast cancer.[22] And that sounds frightening; but in reality, it was a very small risk in the group that had both oestrogen and the progestin. How can a 26 per cent increase be a small risk, you ask?

The five-year follow-up showed 166 cases of breast cancer in the active treatment group of around 8,000 participants, versus 122 in the 8,000 or so in the placebo group – that's 44 extra cases out of 8,000 or so women in the active treatment arm. Yes, that is 26 per cent more, but it's a very small number of people. The next thing that's important to look at is what they call the 'absolute risk' – the number of people who may experience an event in relation to the population at risk. The study found that the number of extra cases per 10,000 person-years (that is, if you watched 10,000 people for a year) that could be attributed to the combined treatment with oestrogen and the progestin (medroxyprogesterone acetate) were seven more cases of coronary heart disease, eight more strokes, eight more pulmonary embolisms, and eight more invasive breast cancers. There were also six fewer colorectal cancers and five fewer hip fractures.[23] There wasn't a lot of mention of the benefits, though.

To put that into perspective, for every 1,000 women aged 50–59 who have a BMI over 30 there are an additional 24 cases of breast cancer above the 23 cases that would normally occur in that population. So, if you take the 44 out of 8,000 or so and break it down, the number of cases per 1,000 is about 5.5 extra, which is about the same as drinking 2 units or more of alcohol a day for those 50–59 years old.[24] A sobering thought, perhaps.

But nothing screams 'good headline' more than '26% increase in breast cancer!' To be fair, these are difficult concepts to get across and you really do need a hand puppet show to help explain if, like me, you aren't mathematically inclined – but that doesn't happen in a busy newsroom. You don't have the benefit of a doctor or a statistician sitting at the end of the newsroom bench to say – 'hang on a sec, let me put that into perspective for you'. Had that been made clearer in the press release though, things may have been very different and a lot of pain saved over the next two decades – but there were way more serious problems with these studies than a poorly worded press release.

It was later found that they were flaws in the design[25] – the average age of the women who were given the MHT was 63 – much older than the usual starting age and a good decade or more past the average age of menopause which is around 51 in most Western countries. And even though two thirds of the participants were over the age of 60, the results of the whole cohort was generalised to all women. And, because they were older, some aged up to 79, their age and their comorbidities put them at higher risk of heart disease and cancer from the outset. And, if all that weren't enough, there were problems with their calculations as a 2006 re-analysis showed – it claimed the increased risk of breast cancer was at just 8 cases per 10,000 person-years and heart disease at 6/10,000 – and that they were not statistically significant, which basically means the extra cases may not have been caused by the MHT.[26]

But the damage was done and to this day the claims that MHT causes cancer still prove hard to quash – especially as the results are often extrapolated beyond conugated equine estrogen and medroxy-progesterone acetate to all the newer and more commonly used transdermal forms of MHT, such as the gels, sprays and patches which are synthesised from yams and soy and are much closer to what the body produces itself than its pregnant mare's pee predecessor.

As the author of the re-analysis wrote: 'The final consequences of these incorrect conclusions are yet to be determined, but it is likely that an untold number of women will suffer from diseases which post-menopausal hormone treatment could have prevented.'

So, now we've established why toilets across the globe were simultaneously flushing – but just how much did they flush? If you go by the effect on prescribing rates – a lot, because those plummeted. In 1994 around 21 per cent of women aged 40–64 in the UK were on hormone therapy, a ten-fold increase since 1987, data shows.[27] But after the release of the study, rates dropped 'precipitously' – by around 50 per cent.[28] In the US, the decline was 46 per cent and 28 per cent in Canada.[29]

In 2022 the UK estimated around 15 per cent of women aged 45–64 were using it.[30] It went on to say that the prescription rate had risen rapidly over the previous two years from 11 per cent, but even 15 per cent is still quite a way off of the 21 per cent from 30 years ago.

In the US the picture is even starker. According to a 2024 article in the *Journal of the American Medical Association* (*JAMA*) 'its estimated use among postmenopausal women declined from about 27% to about 5% from 1999 to March 2020'.[31] Given around 30 per cent of women report severe symptoms, a further 30 per cent have moderate symptoms and as many as 80 per cent have vasomotor symptoms[32] that can last seven years or so on average, it seems we are a long way short of over-treating or over-medicalising. It's a point not lost on Dr Louise Newson, GP, author and podcaster who now also conducts her own research. She says, 'It's concerning that HRT prescribing rates are still alarmingly low – around half of what they were 20 years ago – while women are often prescribed the wrong treatments, such as antidepressants, painkillers, and sleeping tablets, instead of receiving proper care for their menopause symptoms.'

But the menoposse weren't the only ones who called out *The Lancet* series. Two leading Australian doctors and researchers, endocrinologist Professor Susan Davis AO and gynaecologist Professor Rodney Baber co-wrote a scathing rebuttal that was published by the Australasian Menopause Society. They said it was 'disappointing' that *The Lancet* series stated 'that "the principles of health empowerment have not been applied to menopause" when empowerment of women to best navigate their menopause . . . has been the focus of national and international organisations . . . for many years'.[33] They went on to say that in cautioning against 'over-medicalisation', *The Lancet* authors 'seem determined to minimise the important role of MHT in helping many women as they reach menopause. They ignore other published systematic reviews which all agree that MHT is the most effective treatment for vasomotor symptoms, [and] is as effective as other bone-specific therapies (antiresorptive agents) in reducing postmenopausal osteoporosis and associated fractures.'

It's probably fair to say that the series was not universally well received. I asked *The Lancet* for a response twice on why they published the series as it was, and why they didn't publish the response from Haver et al., but received no reply.

In the meantime, back over on social media, things were hotting up with some doctors starting to challenge what had now become the mainstream narrative on the benefits of MHT. Seeing all of these claims and counterclaims play out on a crowded social media feed left a lot of people feeling confused and angry, and some of the doctors who put their heads above the parapet with an argument that runs counter to what popular menopause doctors were saying drew serious fire from those who didn't like what they were now being told.

An example of this are claims that testosterone is good for boosting energy levels, brain fog, muscle mass and overall wellbeing. When one of the world's leading researchers on testosterone in menopause posted that the evidence so far did not support these claim the responses were:

> This is disinformation and misinformation at its best example!

Another followed up with:

> How about you listen to the countless women who are using it and feeling better and let them decide . . . Sometimes I think doctors get so wrapped up in the formalities of it and just want the credit of their name on a damn paper.

And then there's this, taking the argument to new heights – or lows:

> Who gives a shit about your studies . . . Gen X women are tired of waiting and would rather try and see for ourselves and we should be allowed to!

It's a far cry from when pioneers in menopause on social media picked up on the grassroots conversations taking place on Facebook and Instagram more than a decade ago. Dr Newson started her Instagram feed way back in 2016. Her first post was her logo which got eight likes. As of June 2025, she had more than 700,000 followers and her posts attract tens of thousands of views. While there are those who may not agree with her views, you cannot deny her role in propelling the menopause movement forward. She says, her work aims to 'empower people to make informed choices about their health' and when she started her messages resonated with many women who felt they'd been gaslit or hadn't been taken seriously by their own doctor (see Chapter 4). She shot to fame fast with numerous TV appearances and quotes in newspaper articles, because women felt like they were being heard. At last someone cared and understood.

Professor of Endocrinology in Manchester and author of *The Complete Guide to the Menopause*, Dr Annice Mukherjee has been on social media since 2019 and remembers how collegiate the space was back then. But over time she noticed more and more posts that weren't quite factually correct so she started to question the misinformation narratives and paid a heavy price. The space had become black and white – there was no room for nuance.

'I started challenging it. I received a lot of hate on social media, and I thought, "What do I do?" And I realised questioning the sources of misinformation wasn't going to help.' She says the reason for the strong beliefs forming around menopause misinformation involves something called 'confirmation bias'. 'If you're repeatedly seeing convincing rhetoric on social media that says, for example "MHT or testosterone is going to change your life" – that will positively impact your experience. You get both a clinical and a type of incredible enlightening effect. Some people start treatment and think, "Oh my God, it's a miracle". They feel incredible. And those people want to share their experience and believe in the miracle. But most women don't experience that, and no research suggests miraculous effects. And that's the power of the brain.'

Feeling the backlash, she stopped challenging it. 'I just started sharing general information and lifestyle. I found it very difficult to post to counteract misinformation. I still find it very difficult. Sometimes I post things based on unchallengeable facts and I still get hate.'

It's not only the public who attack doctors publicly, the doctors have started attacking each other. The term 'stitch incoming' is a popular one, where someone will take a portion of someone's video and then impose themselves over it or tag another video onto it and then tell you what was wrong with what the other person said. The stitch is meant to represent stitching something together but in these cases it's often more like stitching someone up.

This professional mudslinging has left women thinking, as one wrote:

> These online spats between physicians who are all trying to help women are unhelpful. Surely you guys can try and see links and agreements. Acknowledge possible positives and work together.

Another simply wrote:

Who do I listen to?

It's a worrying trend, Diane Danzebrink says. 'I don't like to see medical health professionals jousting on social media because, ultimately, I don't think it's helpful for the woman who is trying to seek information and help for herself, or her family members, her partner, etc. But I think the problem is that the genie is out of the bottle, and it ain't going back anytime soon.'

One popular UK-based influencer, Cathy Proctor, who has been documenting her menopause journey on Instagram for many years, says she just doesn't know who to believe or trust now.

I've been in the social media menopause community for four and a half years now. When I first started my page in September 2020, it was to share all I had learnt in the previous six months, after stumbling into being perimenopausal (a word I had never heard of before) and frustrated at how I had got to the age of 52 and yet been so unprepared. I was even more confused and upset when it became so apparent after talking to girlfriends, my sisters and anyone else that would listen that it wasn't just me – they also had little knowledge, and any knowledge they did have was based on myth and untruths – mostly from the Women's Health Initiative (WHI) report back in 2002.

In 2020 it felt like safe space, a place where women supported women and a good place to turn to for information that wasn't readily available in the places it should have been – namely doctor surgeries. I felt confident in my decision-making about my own journey and felt confident signposting women to places I felt would help them to educate themselves with factual evidence-based information. But as time has gone on, particularly in this last year, I feel it has become a confusing space. Even specialists are now disagreeing and openly arguing on social media, adding to confusion.

I have gone from someone who felt empowered and knowledgeable and wanted to share all I was learning to help others, including sharing my own story, to now not knowing who to turn to for factual information and feeling confused about my own journey with HRT, let alone trying to help others navigate theirs.

Dr Mukherjee believes she's seeing a slow change as the pendulum starts to swing back to a more central position, but thinks it will take a good few years for women to realise how to navigate social media menopause misinformation. But she's concerned there's a bigger picture here that threatens the system to its heart. If people hold tight to what the popular doctors claim and it doesn't match with the current evidence-based guidelines, women lose trust in the NHS, their doctors and the medical establishment, and that will be hard to win back. She's also concerned that the way menopause is portrayed is scaring younger women. 'The next generation of women heading for menopause are terrified of it. That's a big problem, and I don't want that, because if you go into it terrified, if you're catastrophising about something, it makes the experience worse' and it may not necessarily be that way.

Then there's the FOMO – fear of missing out. 'They ask "Should I be really, really worried about menopause?" "I'm really fit and have no symptoms, but should I be taking HRT anyway?" If you get symptoms, or if you've got osteoporosis or osteopenia, then that's different, you've got a reason to take it, but now everyone feels they have to be on it even if they don't need it or don't want to be on it,' Mukherjee says.

So where does the truth lie? How much do we really know about menopause? And, if you're now more confused than you were before, what can you do to find what's right for you? Don't be disheartened – there have been some positives here which we'll tackle next, while Part 3 covers why managing menopause matters to your long-term health.

2

A hot and sweaty mess

At this point, we're probably all thinking, surely menopause is one thing we should all be able to agree on? After all, it's not just about getting through perimenopause, it's about our long-term health – all those silent changes that we don't see that affect our heart, brain, bones, bladder and beyond. So, why are we arguing? But all is not lost. This democratisation of information does have its upsides.

Associate Professor of Reproductive Health at University College London, obstetrician and gynaecologist and a menopause trainer accredited by the British Menopause Society (BMS), Vikram Talaulikar says it's had a huge impact on the way he practises.

It has changed massively, and largely for the good. And the reason I say that is before social media for menopause or women's health in general, it was a one-way dialogue. Patients were seen by their GP, they'd listen to what their GP said – evidence-based or not; then were referred to a specialist clinic, and they listened to the specialist – evidence-based or not. Most did not have a lot of choice in what they were actually receiving at the other end. They agreed to the instructions given to them about their treatments and the diagnosis made. Even if they wanted to carry out some research on their own there was very little out there which they could easily access because it was all largely stuck in the medical literature, medical textbooks, journals, and online resources that the majority never had access to.

So, there was an element of blind faith in many cases and individuals just got on with it. That's massively changed. You cannot do that now in current medical practice. And a big credit for this goes to social media because most women are now better informed about their condition before they walk through the clinic door. Almost every woman who comes through my clinic door is now aware about what she will likely be offered. She can anticipate in advance what I'm going to tell her about various clinical scenarios, diagnosis, and management, and she's already made a bit of a choice in her mind about which one she will go for – that is a massive improvement. Women can now actively question me if

I give them a different diagnosis or a different scenario. That doesn't mean I'm wrong, but she can question me about why I think A and not B. If I offer five treatment options she can ask me where is the sixth? She would never have known in the past. It's now a two-way discussion and that is amazing.

This is still very much a Western phenomenon though. If I go to a clinic in a less resourced country, this mostly wouldn't happen. Most times, menopause would not be a top health priority. I would be expected to give a diagnosis or my opinion to the woman and she would walk away with her diagnosis and any medications that have been offered without further questions or discussions. That still happens in most of the under-resourced world. So, individuals in the West have benefitted due to social media.

But it's not without a cost. When the patient shows up armed with information that may not be evidence-based or in line with current best practice, things can go horribly wrong. Over the years I've spoken with many, many practitioners who say they are now having to spend much more time in a consultation explaining why something that someone has heard on social media is not necessarily correct.

'This is the negative side of social media,' Talaulikar says. 'If that information is wrong, then it's double work for the clinician. It makes life difficult, because they then believe "you're telling me something wrong". How can a person on social media be wrong – they're telling it to 10,000 or 10 million people. So therein lies the downside to information on social media. If women have had access to wrong information or blurred facts, because of cherry-picked information, and you tell them something different that is evidence-based, they may not accept what you're telling them and you end up in conflict.'

An example he gives is patients who ask for a blood test so they can 'see where they are in their menopause journey' and then, once they've got their blood levels, they can decide how much MHT to take. In practice, blood test results do not determine the dose as blood levels fluctuate regularly across the day so you could end up taking too much or too little. But not all patients will accept that explanation, Talaulikar says, and things go pear-shaped, and it can culminate in complaints being made against the practitioner.

There are two things that come from this that are crucial – trust, and practitioner education. Let's look at trust first. When someone you trust is telling you one thing and someone else is telling you something completely different, you have to make a decision about who you believe. But how? They both say they are experts and they're both citing studies – but who is right? First of all, the answer may not be black and white – there may be a host of nuances that make up the answer. Let's take testosterone and Hyposexual Desire Disorder (HSDD) or low libido, as an example. Testosterone can be prescribed for this, but it doesn't work for everyone, in fact around 40 per cent of women don't respond[1] despite the impression we're given on social media, and that's because libido is multi-faceted. If you no longer find your partner attractive, no amount of testosterone is going to change that. As Chicago-based professor, obstetrician and gynaecologist, author and podcaster with a physical and telehealth practice Dr Lauren Streicher says, we're now into 'husband replacement therapy' (if, of course, your partner is your husband). 'It's true that if you don't like your partner, no drug is going to help, but before you toss him, couple's therapy would be a good first step,' she adds.

The take-home message – even though there is evidence to say it works, it doesn't mean it works for all, all of the time.

A mainstay in establishing trust is understanding the levels of evidence. Sometimes these levels are graded by numbers with 1 being the highest and 7 being the lowest. Often people will hold up a study and say 'this shows X' – and it may well do – but is it a good study? Does it show cause and effect or does it show a link or an association between two things?

Evidence is cumulative. It builds over time as more and more studies show the same thing repeatedly – that is, the findings are replicated time and time again so we know it's not a fluke. At the top of the tree we have what's called a meta-analysis or systematic review. This is where researchers will take as many studies as they can find on a topic, weed out the ones that are poorly done and then look at the good ones that are left and draw a conclusion based on the overall findings. The advantages of that are that you can look at data from many thousands of people which should give a more accurate picture of what the evidence shows to date.

The next level is the randomised controlled trial or RCT. Ideally it should be blinded so no one knows who is getting what treatment, there should be a placebo arm to it (where a sham treatment or sugar pill is given), and it's even better if it's done out of multiple centres so it has a large number and broader pool of participants that better reflect the general population. After that comes a well-designed unrandomised trial, then observational studies that look at de-indentified data from large pools of people that are held by biobanks or insurance company healthcare records, for example. They look for patterns and associations. And moving on down, then come cases studies, and at the bottom of the pile are expert opinions.

The size of studies is important too. A study that is small could show a bias, purely by accident. For example, you might be looking at honey allergies and 6/10 people who you recruited just happen to be allergic, but it would be wrong then to say that 60 per cent of the population is allergic to honey – you need a much bigger study to get a more realistic picture.

Observational studies are popular. They have the advantage of looking at large numbers of people's data, and are often cited as proof of concept. But it's important to remember that while they may show links or correlations between X and Y, they don't show cause and effect. So, they're great for pointing researchers in a direction for future investigations but they're unlikely to change practice because you can't rule out any of the confounding factors or variables that you can't see from the data that could have affected the results.

Opt-in-surveys – which are often done online these days – are also popular but may produce biased results depending on the question asked. In general, you're not likely to answer a survey if the topic doesn't directly affect you. For example, if I do a survey and ask 'I'm looking for people to talk about doctor's management of menopause symptoms', I'm more likely to attract women who've had a poor experience, who think 'yep, I'm answering that one, let me at it!' as they've got something to say and want to see services improved. But if I'd phrased it as 'An evaluation of midlife health management' and asked questions about menopause in it, I'd probably get a very different set of answers. So, it's complicated – but the take-away message is if someone holds up a single study with a handful of people in it and says it shows X = Y and asks 'why aren't they changing the guidelines – look we have proof', you might like to remind them that guidelines are changed based on a large body of accumulated and replicated data. And you will find with virtually every study that you read that they say at the end: 'more research is needed' – it may look like a throw away line, but it is needed. The data gap is real! (See Chapter 5.)

Next, we come to that much-cited phrase 'absence of evidence is not evidence of absence'. Something may not have been studied or may not have been studied adequately to draw a conclusion. This doesn't necessarily mean it won't work or there's been zero effect on anyone, it just means that more work is needed.

It really upsets people when experts say there is no evidence for X because the studies show it didn't work. Again, testosterone is a good example here because anecdotally many people say they have less fatigue, more energy and less brain fog, but as yet the data doesn't bear this out. The result is a chorus of people saying 'well I feel much better', 'it was the icing on the cake for me', and 'why don't you do better studies!' But there are two important points here:

a) some people in the studies may have had these benefits but not enough of them to say 'Eureka, it worked! Let's change the guide-lines and recommend it for everybody with those symptoms!'

b) a study isn't about a single individual; don't take it personally, it's really not about you and your experience, it's about the bigger picture, what happened in large pools of people – the ones you'd look at in a meta-analysis that show repeated results in large groups of people.

As gynaecologist, BBC columnist and Femtech strategist Michelle Griffin explains: 'We've lost the ranking of evidence, and that's not to say all studies needed to come from some top professor in an ivory tower, but it needs to be reproducible, and I think that's the key thing. That's why anecdotal evidence falls down because it's not reproducible. It worked for Sally, it worked for you, but that's not reproducible. And when I put it up and throw it against the wall in a clinical trial, and I take out all the confounding factors, and I need to repeat it time after time, if I haven't got that result, then I haven't got what I thought I was going to have, I've just got a bunch of anecdotes. And maybe this is getting very philosophical, but there has to be a kind of reference, a rule book that we all agree to agree to – a set of good practice principles. Yes, bringing it out of the ivory tower, throw it out for everyone to hear about, to discuss – that's great, but whatever we say has to be backed up, and we have to clearly state whether that backup is good or low-level evidence.'

I often see on social media comments along the lines of 'we can't wait for you to do your studies, we need this NOW!' which are understandable, but everything has risks and benefits, and you want to be sure that your guidelines are based on the best assessment of both. Take a look at Chapter 4 to find out why it's important.

Who do you trust?

We've sorted the evidence, but what about the person you're listening to, or when you're choosing a doctor? Women are often told 'do your own research, your due diligence' – but what are you looking for? Is the number of followers a good indication of the quality of their information, or is it their ability to tell a good story? Is it a good review, or is it that they represent a certain organisation?

Dr Lauren Streicher has been watching this space blossom over the past few years and has some good tips on who to trust when you're picking a doctor:[2]

1 Your doctor doesn't have to have a vagina to treat you. There are some amazing male doctors who treat menopause very well, so if you're comfortable with a man, their gender shouldn't be an issue. (Some people have said it's better to see a woman as they'll be more empathetic and who wants a man mansplaining menopause to you? But if we apply the opposite logic and say men should only see men for penis problems then female urologists lose out, as do the men who could have been treated by them.)

2 The number of letters they have after their name may not be an indication of their menopause skills – look instead for the number of years they've spent working in menopause or the courses they've done or the societies they are members of (not that the latter automatically confers knowledge, but at least they'll have access to it!) In the US there is no 'board certification' for menopause, she warns. (If you're in the UK, the British Menopause Society has a list

of its accredited menopause practitioners on its website – unfortunately at the time of writing there were only 452 of them. You can ask your GP practice if there is a doctor or nurse who has an interest in women's health and menopause and if not ask to be referred to a menopause specialist. In the US the Menopause Society has a list as well and if you're down under, the Australasian Menopause Society is a good spot to check.)

3 If you are being referred by a hospital in the US – or an insurance company in any country – check the websites or CVs of the doctors that are being recommended because if their primary interest is delivering babies then they may not know all that much about life at the other end of the reproductive cycle. (This happened to me in the UK when I was fortunate enough to have private health insurance for a brief window in time. I was sent a bunch of names for doctors who spent most of their time in obstetrics. Not one of them mentioned menopause as an interest on their websites, so I went back to the company and said 'thank you, but I think I'd be wasting these doctors' time and your money, could you find me someone else on your books who lists menopause as an interest?' and they did. They lump all obstetricians and gynaecologists in the same bucket, and as we know the amount of menopause education a doctor, even a gynaecologist, gets at university is virtually negligible – so you can't rely on them knowing very much unless they've taken the time afterwards to do some extra study.) As Dr Streicher says, if you walk into the waiting room and it's full of pregnant women, you're probably in the wrong place.

4 People who teach medical students as well as practice can be a good choice, she says, because they are highly likely to be up-to-date with the latest research.

5 Don't rely on reviews – you don't know if they're genuine, or from the doctor's mother or a disgruntled patient.

6 Look for red flags on the doctor's website – do they prescribe pellets or compounded hormone therapies? Do they talk about 'hormone balancing', which is not a medically recognised thing – it doesn't exist. Dr Streicher says it's nothing more than a way of pushing expensive and unnecessary tests. Another thing to look for is if they do procedures that aren't covered by insurance or

backed by evidence beyond that delivered by the manufacturer of that treatment? These could signal you may end up paying for a lot of stuff that you don't really need but not getting what you actually do.

Once you've got an appointment, how can you tell if your doctor knows anything about menopause or if you should run a mile? Dr Streicher says there are a couple of good indications here – if they tell you to take black cohosh or stand in front of an open fridge for your hot flushes, or that a glass of wine will help with painful sex and your inability to orgasm, strap those running shoes on and head for the hills.

But how do you even know if what you're experiencing is part of that rocky road towards menopause known as perimenopause? The *Women's Health Strategy* says just 9 per cent of women say they had enough information about menopause let alone its ever-expanding list of symptoms.[3] I've seen some posts saying there are 100 menopause symptoms. It seems to be a bit like a black hole – expanding exponentially to include things like procrastination. (Procrastination, by the way, is not a symptom of menopause – you may decide to put something off and do it later because you can't concentrate or have brain fog, but procrastination itself is not a symptom, it's an outcome from a decision you make.)

Generally, most lists contain around 30–40 or so symptoms so it may surprise you then that the only ones actually associated with menopause, according to a 2025 presentation given for the International Menopause Society (IMS), are:[4]

- Vasomotor symptoms, the hot flushes and night sweats – duvet on, duvet off – very irritating
- Changes to periods in terms of regularity and heaviness
- Mood changes/depression like symptoms
- Vaginal symptoms – the Genitourinary Syndrome of Menopause (GSM) which includes things like dryness, pain during or after sex, bladder leakage and increased frequency of UTIs. These affect up to 85% of women, more commonly in postmenopause (see Chapter 9).
- Sleep disturbances (affect around 45 per cent)

Associated atypical symptoms are considered to be:

- Joint pain
- Palpitations which are experienced by 3–5 per cent

And just to confuse things, if you're like me, you may not have changes to your period until a few months before they finally stop – but boy, was I moody! A large study is being done in Australia by Professor Susan Davis, a world leader in menopause research, to show if many of the other commonly cited symptoms really are associated with menopause or if they're associated with midlife in general. This is especially important because we have many companies offering products or workplace advice but in order for them to be effective or the advice given to be meaningful, they need to be based on evidence (see Chapter 6).

Is it always menopause? Why has my doctor sent me for so many other tests?

Many aeons ago I worked as the editor of a brand-new NHS-style website for consumers in Australia. To launch we had to have 240 'conditions' ready to go with definitions of what they were, the causes, the symptoms, the diagnoses and the treatments. I commissioned them, edited them and sent them off to be medically reviewed for accuracy before publishing them. It was an eye opener in many ways because it became apparent very quickly just how many conditions have virtually identical symptoms. (It was also a great cure for hypochondria because I realised very quickly that I couldn't have all of these, but it also made me realise just how tricky it can be for a GP to work out what it is that you've got – so show them some love.) For example, menopause symptoms can overlap considerably with many other conditions like thyroid or auto-immune conditions or even anaemia (see table ahead). This is why your GP may order blood tests or refer you on to rule out other causes. Menopause may be offered as a one stop answer for all ills, and that might be the right call, but you'd be pretty unhappy if your doctor missed any of these other ones. And in some cases, you could have a combination of things going on simultaneously.

Symptoms	Menopause	Thyroid condition (hyper and hypo)	Heart condition	Autoimmune conditions	Sleep apnoea	Anaemia
Fatigue	x	x	x	x	x	x
Weight gain	x	x		x		
Hair loss	x	x		x		x
Anxiety	x	x		x		
Night sweats/hot flushes	x	x	x	x		
Palpitations	x	x	x	x		x
Dry/itchy skin	x	x		x		
Headaches	x	x		x		x
Joint pain/ muscle stiffness or aches	x	x		x		
Dizziness/ light-headed	x	x	x	x	x	x
Vaginal dryness	x	x		x		
Memory issues/brain fog	x	x		x		
Insomnia	x	x		x	x	x
Irregular periods	x	x		x		
Irritability	x	x		x	x	
Low libido	x	x		x	x	

Of course, this is nowhere near the full list of symptoms that are associated with menopause. Others include tinnitus (ringing in the ears), bleeding gums, dry mouth and dry eyes, bloating, flatulence, new or worsening allergies, bladder leakage and incontinence, prolapses, frozen shoulders, panic attacks, a feeling like ants crawling under your skin (called formication – not to be confused with fornication which would probably be a lot more fun), cold flashes, brittle nails, sore boobs, strange electrical zapping sensations and tingling extremities – and it goes on. Again, many of these may have other causes so it's always wise to get things checked out thoroughly.

Mind the gap – in knowledge

Now you could be forgiven for thinking your doctor should be an expert on menopause and that they'd teach it at med school; after all, women make up around 50 per cent of the global population and every one of us who lives long enough will go through it – but you'd be sadly mistaken. A freedom of information request by Diane Danzebrink's Menopause Support in 2021 revealed that a staggering 41 per cent of the 32 UK-based medical schools who responded did not have a mandatory menopause education programme for their students.[5] This means some doctors may leave university with no education in menopause at all. Two universities didn't appear to know if they had a course, which is truly comforting because clearly they have no idea of what's in their curriculum. One university responded saying it wasn't mandatory but 'students are expected to engage'. What exactly they were expected to engage in wasn't made clear.

Seven universities delivered one hour's worth of education, one offered seven hours and Edinburgh offered around ten – so hats off to Edinburgh. For the others, the general expectation was that students would gain experience in their rotations with GPs or obstetrics and gynaecology. But there are some problems with relying on this:

a) they may not see any or enough women to gain any useful insights
b) it relies on the attitudes of the doctor or gynaecologist they are training with – and if they're still telling their patients that taking 'MHT is postponing the inevitable' (as mine in the UK did), or 'they don't believe in it', or 'it'll give you cancer' as I've heard from other women, then those students aren't really going to be getting a lot of useful information.

And it's a similar picture in the US. There are loads of videos on social media of gynaecologists, urologists and others saying they were given virtually no education on menopause when they were at university, and those claims are backed up by studies that looked at how much (or how little) menopause education American doctors in residence had received. Back in 2019 the Mayo Clinic surveyed doctors in residency programs across the US. A total of 183 trainees responded with most saying they thought menopause education was important, but the researchers identified gaps in their competency with just over a third (34.4 per cent) saying they wouldn't offer hormone therapy to menopausal women with symptoms even if they had no contraindications and only 38.7 per cent said they would prescribe it up to the average age of menopause to women who had gone through premature menopause. Just over 20 per cent of 177 respondents who answered questions on education said they hadn't received any lectures on menopause and only 12 of them (6.8 per cent) felt adequately prepared to manage women experiencing menopause.[6] Skipping ahead to 2022 and not a lot had changed. A survey of 99 US-based ob-gyn residents found that while 92.9 per cent strongly agreed there was a need for a standardised menopause curriculum, only 31.3 per cent had received any menopause education at all. On the upside, at least one in three of them who did get some education spent some time in a menopause clinic. But as the researchers concluded, 'menopause education and resources vary across residency programs, with the majority lacking a dedicated menopause curriculum.'[7] So, we still have some way to go.

Much of this may be due to the results of the Women's Health Initiative study that made MHT such a toxic topic that it was no longer on the table for discussion. And if it were, the chorus line was, until recently, 'don't touch it'. The result? Consumers often feel they are now more informed and up to date than their own doctor due to the information they've got from the influencers they listen to. And then they think they aren't being listened to.

'This is what I tell everyone,' Mary Claire Haver says. 'Your patients are getting their information from social media – good and bad – and they're just going to take up more time in a visit.' Her suggestion, don't get frustrated, but 'acknowledge that if you're going to practice menopause care you need to upskill your own knowledge base'.

But upskilling is a controversial topic. You would have hoped that with all the talk about menopause over the past few years that doctors would be on top of it by now – but it seems not. A 2023 survey of 20 menopausal women, 30 family doctors and 10 gynaecologists funded by the pharmaceutical company Besins showed that the doctors held considerable differences in their beliefs and attitudes towards menopause and the practitioners often showed 'a lack of confidence in prescribing HRT'. Because of this secondary care services can be 'overwhelmed by an explosion in uncomplicated referrals which could be effectively managed in primary care'. It concluded, not surprisingly, that there are 'multiple opportunities to address these gaps in knowledge, including the use of HCP [healthcare professional] education'.[8]

This may go some way towards explaining why a 2024 survey of 1,500 women by Mumsnet found that 40 per cent of women didn't trust their family doctor to manage their menopause.[9]

You would expect after the litany of ongoing stats that have literally filled pages on multiple reports that that have recommended mandatory catch up education for doctors, and the calls from multiple advocacy groups, that it would be a 'no brainer' and be instigated post-haste. It would even save money (see Chapter 5). But again, you'd be sadly disappointed. The UK government has rejected a recommendation calling for it claiming that it's not within its remit to dictate what should be taught to doctors and it believes the Royal College of General Practitioners (RCGP) when it says it's got it sorted.[10] The above stats would beg to differ, as would a coroner in Somerset in the UK called Samantha Marsh who in May 2025 issued a *Prevention of Future Deaths* report to the RCGP and NHS England, among others, calling for them to take action on GP training or explain why they wouldn't. Her call followed an inquest into the death of Jacqueline Anne Potter who drove her car into the path of an oncoming truck. The coroner said her menopause symptoms had contributed to her death.[11]

The Australian government has taken a similar stance in its response to the recommendations from the Senate inquiry into menopause and perimenopause.[12] It has, however, put AU$1.5 million into a three-year incentivisation programme to help get doctors enrolled in menopause continuing professional development courses. It's a small step in the right direction, but clearly there's a disconnect somewhere here.

The advantages of having a well-educated medical workforce, it's argued, are that it would ultimately reduce health costs because many of the problems that were previously dealt with individually could be quickly solved and waiting rooms would be far less clogged with what Haver said were described as 'whining women' during her training – the patients who turned up with a long list of disparate complaints that had no obvious cause. (And if you think that's bad, a doctor in the UK told me files at her training hospital were marked with 'FFF': fat, fifties, female – let that sink in for a second!)

In the US, Jennifer Weiss-Wolf has joined forces with a group of vocal practitioners including Haver to produce a 'Citizen's Guide to Menopause Advocacy'. Among its six action points is 'Update and Mandate Education for [healthcare] Providers' and it gives women the information they need to contact their state or federal representatives to demand change.

And change can happen. Due to the consistent advocacy of grass-roots groups like Danzebrink's and her Make Menopause Matter campaign, menopause was added to the school curriculum in 2019 and also to medical schools from 2024, but we don't know as yet exactly what that curriculum looks like.

The rise of the menopause coach

The lack of information on menopause, but the desire for it, and the need for help and support has spawned a new set of service providers – the menopause coach, menopause workplace coach, the menopause dietician, menopause nutritionist, menopause fitness coach, menopause doulas – I could go on. And there are a huge number of pluses to this because you can now access an array of information and services with the click of a button. But of course there's another side too. How do we know if the information they are presenting is accurate or if it's aligned to the products, diet plans or exercise programmes they may be selling? And once again, what do we really know about their credentials?

Dieticians should have a university degree and be registered to practice. For nutritionists you would expect that they would have done a degree or a course from a recognised academic institution. For fitness coaches in the UK you'd expect that they will have a degree in exercise physiology/sports science or at least have done an accredited Level 3 or 4 training programme.

For 'menopause coaches' or 'workplace champions', many will say they've done an accredited menopause course, but I just want to give you a small word of warning about 'accredited courses'. A CPD accredited course is not an indication of quality content or high standards.

How do I know this? Because I have registered menopause courses for doctor education for the Menopause Research and Education Fund. You submit a form to show there are learning modules with outcomes, but the person assessing that has absolutely zero idea about menopause or the quality or accuracy of the information that will be taught. All they want to know is if it's clearly set out with learning objectives. There are loads of these menopause courses on the market ranging from as little as £29 to almost £1,000, so if you are thinking of doing one, try and find one that is run by someone with medical experience and an interest/qualification in menopause, or a background in psychology or counselling. But that information may be harder to find than you'd think.

A quick search of the offerings online provides some truly scary results. Some coaching courses teach you about 'estrogen dominance' or 'hormone balancing' – these are not medically accepted terms. Others teach you about the benefits of progesterone cream. These creams are not recommended as progesterone is not absorbed well through the skin, so if you are relying on that for endometrial protection, or advising others to use it, that could be dangerous for their future health.[13] (Just before you say 'but hang on, it's in my patches' – they use a progestin, most commonly norethisterone, not progesterone, and it's not in a cream.) Others offer courses that last just 40 minutes. Many of the ones I looked at don't say what the qualifications are of those who have pulled the courses together except that they have 'years of experience'. And some of them aren't cheap – they're charging about the same as the British Menopause Society charges medical practitioners for its course.

Where does that leave you if you're looking for a coach? Danzebrink advises that, if you're going to spend money on services from these providers, 'ask them "what are your qualifications to do this? What's your experience in this space?" Because it's all very well having qualifications but if you've got no experience working in the space, and if you've done an online course for £35, well, that doesn't mean that you've got any experience helping people. One of the things that has become an issue is that if somebody has had an experience of menopause themselves, and it's been a poor experience, they think, "oh, I want to help other people". That's great that they want to help other people, but we always have to remember that one individual's experience of menopause doesn't translate to other people's and doing a £35 weekend course certainly doesn't make you knowledgeable and it certainly doesn't make you an expert.'

The other thing to keep an eye out for is people who use 'I'm a member of the British Menopause Society' or 'affiliated with the British Menopause Society' or any of the other menopause societies as a credential. I am a member of the British Menopause Society, the International Menopause Society and the Menopause Society – but all that means is I've paid my fees as a non-medically qualified member and I can access the journals and other information. It doesn't make me a menopause expert. It's not a qualification. So, as they say, *caveat emptor*; buyer beware.

3

The thing about menopause . . .

I was talking to an old friend recently who said she'd been to see a dermatologist and had asked him if her itchy skin could be related to menopause. He'd told her that it might be, but went on to say that from an evolutionary stand point she really shouldn't be here at all (itchy or otherwise) because 'women should not live long enough to experience menopause'. After I picked my jaw up off the floor, I thought to myself 'are we really still at this point?' and resolved that it was time to have a good look at some of the prevailing myths, misconceptions and theories that abound about menopause, and where possible, set the record straight. These are important, because the way we view menopause influences the way we approach or treat it. There are anthropological theories and then there are our beliefs or opinions based on what we deem to be 'natural' or 'unnatural'. Either way, as we know, almost everyone has an opinion on why menopause happens and what we should or shouldn't do about it.

First of all, let's look at what menopause is. I know most people will know this so I'll keep it brief. The word menopause refers to the end of your periods. It may surprise you to hear that the term only came into existence in 1821, but there seems to be confusion over who said it first with some saying it was coined by French physician Charles-Pierre-Louis de Gardanne, who blended the word *men* – meaning 'month' in Greek – with *pausis*, which means 'to cease or stop'. Others say it was another physician called Charles Negrier. Either way, it means your ovaries have stopped producing ova or eggs so your uterus no longer needs to prepare a nice lining for a fertilised egg to embed in and grow a baby. The shedding of this lining every month is your period.

Menopause is one point of time in your life and it is a retrospective diagnosis generally made 12 months after your last period. (I say generally, because if you're under 40 they may wait 24 months. And remember, contraception is still required if it's important for you.) You are then said to have 'gone through' menopause. In the UK and many other countries you are then referred to as postmenopausal, and this is how you are for the rest of your life. In the US some people simply call it menopausal.

The period before you hit menopause, or it hits you as some would say, is called perimenopause. During this time your hormone levels are simultaneously declining and fluctuating like crazy and you may experience various symptoms related to menopause, the classic ones being low mood, changes to periods (heavy, lighter, more or less frequent) and the vasomotor symptoms (hot flushes and night sweats, or chills.) These can start a few years or so before your periods stop and may continue well afterwards as well. On average it's said that vasomotor symptoms can last on average 7.4 years[1] but some women experience them into their 80s and there are differences between ethnic groups with Black and Hispanic women having them for longer than White or Asian women.

The thing is, we are all unique in our menopause journey. Some people will 'sail through' barely noticing it, while around 30 per cent of people will have moderate symptoms and another 30 per cent will have severe symptoms. These can interfere with sleep, wreak havoc on mental health and/or mood, or cause brain fog to the point that they just can't function properly at work. People often say they think they're going mad or developing dementia and the impact on productivity and the economy can be considerable and costly (see Chapter 5).

The average age that women go through menopause in high income countries is around 51 (range 45–55). In low income or developing countries it can be a few years earlier, around 48. If you go through menopause between the ages of 40–44 it's called early menopause, and this affects about one in ten women. If you go through menopause under the age of 40 it's called Premature Ovarian Insufficiency, or POI, and this affects somewhere between 3.5–5 per cent of the global population.[2,3] The rate is higher in developing countries than it is in high-income countries where it's said to be around 1 per cent of the population.

So, let's hit one myth on the head straightaway: when someone says you're too young to be going through menopause, they're wrong – you can never be too young to go through menopause. It may not be as common, but it happens. In fact, some women never even have a period – they are menopausal in their teens and their stories are particularly harrowing as more often than not they aren't diagnosed until much later, so have no idea of what they're going through at the time. They're left wondering why they can't concentrate at school, why they're having hot flushes and irrational moods, only to be faced later with the reality that they will never be able to naturally conceive, which can be devastating for some.

I listened to Sheree Hargraves, a campaigner for POI awareness, at a conference describing how she went through this in her teens. When the doctor told her she was in menopause, he handed her a pamphlet where the faces of 50-year-old women stared back at her. She said it was impossible to relate and she felt isolated and alone.

Over the years I've interviewed a number of young women like her and they've described how they had to pretend to be having periods at school so they'd fit in. They'd buy tampons and go to the loo to pretend to change them. Later they had difficulties having sex due to vaginal dryness, which affected their relationships, as did finding the 'right time' to tell a new partner you can't have children. When do you do that – the first date, or do you wait until the relationship has formed only to risk them walking out the door? (There is an excellent book by Dr Siobhan O'Sullivan called *My Life on Pause* that describes exactly this dilemma and how it affected her and her relationships as she went through POI in her late 20s/early 30s.)

But these are not the only challenges, premature menopause puts them at greater risk of developing heart disease, cognitive issues including dementia and osteoporosis because they've lost the protective effects of oestrogen that the majority of us have until our 50s. Having access to MHT is vital for them, unless contradicted due to an oestrogen-positive cancer for example, until the age of average menopause. So, timely diagnosis and support is crucial. (Charities like the Daisy Network in the UK provide support if this has affected you or someone you know, and an excellent book on this is *The Complete Guide to POI and Early Menopause* by Drs Mandy Leonhardt and Hannah Short, which is very practical and supportive.)

How is menopause diagnosed?

In the 45-plus age group the diagnosis is based on symptoms. You do not need a blood test to diagnose it but your doctor may do some other tests to confirm your symptoms are menopause related and to rule out other things that may have similar symptoms such as a thyroid condition.

My doctor did do some tests including checking my thyroid function and Follicle Stimulating Hormone (FSH) just to be sure. FSH, as its name suggests, is a hormone that stimulates an ovary to produce an egg. If it's above normal levels, it's an indication that it's having to work hard to make that happen and you may be heading towards menopause or in menopause.

In my case, there was no doubt about where I was. Now, bear in mind I had known my GP for many years, and we got on very well. I had been away for a few years living in Russia and had come home to get my fingerprints taken for my UK visa – don't ask! Anyway, he decided to do a battery of tests since it had been a while since anything had been looked at and threw the FSH in too after I'd told him I was more snappy and less tolerant than usual. (He expressed sympathy for my family.) When the results came back, he said, and I quote, 'Jesus Christ . . . talk about trying to flog a dead horse!' My FSH was sky high and my ovaries were flatlining.

Just to be clear – you don't normally need this test if you're over 45 unless you have atypical symptoms.[4]

If you're in perimenopause, the oestrogen levels are constantly fluctuating so measuring them isn't going to give you a great indication of where you are. They could be high at the point when the blood is taken so may give a false indication of where you're at, so it's recommended that symptoms are used as a guide to diagnosis. If you are under 45, clinicians may do a blood test to look at your FSH. Again, taking blood samples of your oestrogen and progesterone levels isn't generally recommended as it may not give you an accurate picture of where you are in your menopause journey because the levels are fluctuating throughout the day.

If you are under 40, the UK's NICE guidelines on menopause[5] recommend that two blood tests for FSH level are taken 4–6 weeks apart. Newer international guidelines are suggesting one FSH test and a history of irregular or no periods.[6] Please note this is a very brief summary of the diagnosis guidelines. Please see the references if you want to know more about these. The guidelines do not recommend routinely using a test called an anti-Müllerian hormone test to diagnose Premature Ovarian Insufficiency. This test gives an indication of the number of eggs left and may be useful for fertility treatments as it gives an idea of how well the ovaries will respond to stimulation to produce eggs, but it is not regarded as a useful or reliable predictor of menopause.

There are other causes of menopause too. Certain medications can cause menopause as can some cancer treatments, like chemotherapy. Menopause from chemo may not be permanent, but for some people it can be. Surgical menopause occurs when the ovaries are removed and it's called a bilateral oophorectomy. It often goes hand in hand with a hysterectomy – when your uterus is removed. If the fallopian tubes are taken as well, the surgery is called a bilateral salpingo-oophorectomy – a name that rolls off the tongue.

Whether it's chemical, medical or surgical, you'll be plunged into menopause and the effects can be devastating, especially on mental health. Menopause advocate Diane Danzebrink knows this only too well. She had her ovaries removed but unfortunately was not given the right advice or follow-up support after her operation and very quickly found herself in a very dark place. In her book *Making Menopause Matter* she describes how she lost confidence overnight, became crippled with anxiety and increasingly irrational.

'I had fallen off the edge of a cliff into a dark abyss with no way out where each day felt darker than the last,' she wrote. 'I felt useless, hopeless and worthless. I had no idea where the real me had disappeared to; I had lost my joy . . . I was a husk of the woman that I used to be.'

In a paragraph that makes me cry every time I read it, she wrote, 'One morning, several months after my surgery, I woke from another torturous night filled with anxiety and panic. I got up and looked out of the window onto what felt like an increasingly dark and scary world and thought to myself: this is my life now, I can't do this anymore.' Later that day she tried to drive her car into the path of an oncoming truck, but fortunately 'a little dog called Henry saved my life'. From the back seat of her car, he barked as she went to swerve into its path and she stopped. She couldn't take the dog with her.

When she got home Diane told her husband and they spoke to the doctor. She was given MHT and, slowly, the lights came back on. She vowed that no one should go through what she'd gone through and has successfully advocated for better education, information and treatment for menopausal women ever since, and I'm proud to call her a friend and inspiration and trustee of the Menopause Research and Education Fund (MREF). Research she's done shows just how poorly treated women who go through surgical menopause are after their operations (see Chapter 4).

For the vast majority of women, though, menopause is a 'natural' occurrence – something all those born with ovaries will go through at some stage. But as menopause's moment has blossomed to a movement and the calls to have its symptoms taken seriously and treated (if need be) have grown, so too has the backlash, with articles popping up regularly in the media featuring women proclaiming they sailed through, so what's wrong with this generation of snowflakes? It's natural, they state, it's what you're meant to go through – a rite of passage like childbirth, and you'll be wiser and better off for it when you get 'to the other side'.

Now, there's a lot to break down in here so I'll take these points one by one.

It's natural

The *Cambridge Dictionary* defines 'natural' as: 'found in nature and not involving anything made or done by people'. By that term, yes, menopause is natural (unless induced). But just because something is natural doesn't mean that it doesn't cause symptoms that some people may need, or wish, to have relieved.

This was a point made clearly on social media by GP, author and menopause specialist Dr Naomi Potter. She posted that no one should feel 'shamed out' of starting MHT because those around you say 'it's natural, you don't need it'.

She argued some diseases occur 'naturally' in your body, but you wouldn't decide not to treat them. Equally you wouldn't choose not to get glasses for your declining eyesight or hearing aids for your hearing loss – both of which can occur 'naturally' as we age.

This is not to say that menopause is a 'disease', 'deficiency' or 'condition' that 'needs treating', but she argues that women should not be shamed or guilted out of seeking help if they need it – but they are. In her practice she regularly hears women saying they were embarrassed to seek help as their friends saw it as a sign of weakness so they'd tried to 'tough it out' for as long as they could. Others have told her they'd never tell their friends that they've decided to start taking MHT because of the judgemental opinions.

I reposted this post because I agree with it. If you have symptoms and feel that your quality of life is affected, then you should be entitled to seek help for them without incurring the wrath or opinions of others. You don't have to 'tough it out' and no one is going to give you a reward for it. After posting I felt the heat, with people saying 'How dare I call menopause a disease?' I wasn't, the post was clear, but it shows just how polarised views are.

'We've now reached a place in history where we have these kind of diametrically opposing camps. In one camp everyone should have HRT, and in another camp we have the "No, no, it's a natural occurrence" – you should be able to breathe and wild swim your way through it. And that's not helpful for anybody because ultimately it's a very personal experience. There's probably one million and one ways in between both of those things and you're going to find yourself somewhere on that scale,' Danzebrink says.

Vikram Talaulikar, BMS-accredited menopause specialist, agrees the 'it's natural, so suck it up' argument doesn't hold water – not even freezing cold, wild swimming water! 'You end up at the other extreme where everything is classed as "normal, normal, normal" and they say "no, you should be nowhere near hormones". It's one thing to focus on the positives and how some people can manage with a certain approach, but we need a balanced message and we're not having that right now.'

Mary Claire Haver sums it up well: 'I don't know what other medication apart from weight loss drugs that attracts so many opinions and why there's such a moral price tag applied to hormone therapy and to weight loss medications. It just blows my mind. Every woman may or may not choose hormone replacement therapy, or may or may not be a candidate for hormone replacement therapy, but every woman deserves an informed conversation from an informed provider so she can make a decision for herself.'

No one complained before

There's a lot to unpack here.

No, they may not have complained about menopause per se, but they did complain about a lot of other things. If you grew up in Australia you may be familiar with the saying 'have a cup of tea, a Bex and a good lie down' – the slogan used to advertise a compound of aspirin, phenacetin (a pain reliever) and caffeine that was popular after World War II, particularly in the '50s and '60s, among middle-aged women who were feeling stressed and anxious. It was often called 'mother's little helper' – a term which may have a completely different connotation these days! It was withdrawn from the market in the 1970s when it was discovered that it was addictive and associated with kidney problems.[7]

But it wasn't the only option available for 'unhappy' housewives. By the 1960s, benzodiazepines like Valium were a staple in many Western homes for frazzled midlife women. From 1968–1982 Valium was 'mother's little helper' in the US and was the top-selling drug for anxiety and insomnia with 2 million tablets sold in 1978 alone across the country.[8] The marketing for these tablets was directed straight at at lonely, depressed and anxious middle-aged, menopausal women. One ad featured a fictional teacher called Mrs Raymond who was suffering with 'excessive psychic tension and associated depressive symptoms accompanying her menopause'. But, her pupils did a 'double take' when she re-appeared at school after taking this wonder drug looking 'trim and smartly dressed, the way she was when school began'.

Before Valium there were barbiturates, which had been used for around 100 years for multiple purposes including treating various mental health disorders, epilepsy and as an anaesethesia. They were also prescribed to help with sleep, anxiety and to induce a sense of calm and they were popular. The production of barbiturates in the US increased by more than 400 per cent from 1933 to 1936 when some 70 tons were sold in the US alone. By 1955 they had to produce enough to treat 10 million people annually.[9] But barbiturates had their downside – they were highly addictive. In 1965 it was estimated that there were 135,000 addicts in the UK and 250,000 in the US where 30 pills a day were needed for every person, every year and there were a number of deaths from overdoses attributed to it, including Marilyn Monroe's.

Between the 1940s and 1970s, the collection of maladies that women were suffering from, which reduced them to raging, irrational and/or blithering wrecks, was called 'the housewife's syndrome' or 'housewives' fatigue' and was often put down to the frustration of being a post-war generation who were overly educated but understimulated at home to the point that they were driven to depression and anger. One medical journal in 1964 described it as a 'modern psychosomatic syndrome' – affecting the mind and body, while American feminist and author Betty Friedan called it the 'problem with no name' in her book *The Feminine Mystique*. She called on women to right the injustices of gender inequity so they could 'develop to their fullest potential'. There was no mention of menopause here, possibly for a variety of reasons – it wasn't spoken about and no one knew at that time that rage, tearfulness, anxiety and depression could be associated with perimenopause and menopause.

But, let's face it, women have always been 'trouble', well before we were afforded the luxury of education. The word 'hysteria' comes from the Greek word *hystera* which means 'womb' or 'uterus', and it was believed that this organ wandered around the body causing all sorts of mischief and unseemly symptoms. According to Aretaeus, a second-century physician, it was attracted by pleasant smells but repulsed by 'fetid' ones and moved away. Logically then, the treatment for a runaway womb was 'scent therapy' which would entice it back to its proper position. Not all of his contemporaries agreed with this. One called Soranus wrote, 'the uterus does not issue forth like a wild animal from the lair, delighted by fragrant odours and fleeing bad odours, rather it is drawn together because of stricture caused by inflammation'.[10] Despite his entreaties, the myth of the wandering womb prevailed. Hippocrates, the father of the 'do no harm' philosophy in medicine mentioned it again in the fifth century, and in 1603 it was referred to by English physician Edward Jorden, in his publication 'The Suffocation of the Mother' which was apparently the first English language text on the subject of the wandering womb and hysteria.

By Victorian times, a woman going through the menopause was considered to be emotionally unstable. 'During this "climacteric period", she may well have been prescribed leeching or bloodletting from the ankle. Her doctor would have advised against reading novels, going to parties and dancing. For a 45–50-year-old Victorian woman, an onslaught of instability and madness was considered inevitable', a Royal College of Nurses publication claims.[11] (Those leeches, by the way, were sometimes applied to the vulva, the cervix or the perineum[12] – the area between the vulva and the anus, or even on the anus – depending on the malady. Just let that visual image sink in for a moment! You can thank me later.)

A little later, psychoanalyst Sigmund Freud delivered an unflattering description of the character transformation menopausal women underwent saying they became 'quarrelsome, vexatious and overbearing'.[13] Fortunately for mankind, the discovery of oestrogen was just around the corner.

In the late 1800s, French scientist Claude Bernard showed that glands had internal secretions that could influence other organs. This led, in 1897, to the use of ovarian extracts as a treatment for hot flushes. Then, in 1906, two American scientists, Edward Allen and Edgar Doisy, discovered that secretions from the ovaries influenced 'estrus' – when animals went on heat. From that the term 'estrogen' was born, taken from the Greek word *oistros* (from the bite of a gadfly that apparently made people spring into action and is connected with passion) and *gennan* (which means 'to produce'). It took another 21 years for the hormone to be isolated and a further 17 years for the first synthetic oestrogen product to hit the market. In 1939 it was launched as Premarin®, named after the pregnant mare's urine that it was derived from (premar-in) and in 1942 the FDA approved it to treat hot flushes, mood swings and insomnia associated with menopause. By 1992 it was a bestseller in the United States, and by 1997 sales exceeded $1 billion.[14]

The fountain of youth

To get to that point though it had a good push along. It was hailed as the cure to ageing by the UK-born gynaecologist Robert Wilson, who practised on New York's fashionable Park Avenue. He wrote in his 1966 bestseller *Feminine Forever* that 'the unpalatable truth must be faced that all postmenopausal women are castrates'. Ouch. 'Many physicians simply refuse to recognize menopause for what it is – a serious, painful and often crippling disease,' he went on. But, if they took hormones their problems would be over.

In a statement that rivals Freud's in its distaste for menopausal women's moods he wrote: 'Every woman alive today has the option of remaining feminine forever.' She would no longer need to 'fret about the cruel irony of women aging faster than men'. With hormone therapy her 'breasts and genital organs will not shrivel. She will be much more pleasant to live with and will not become dull and unattractive.' (Well, thank God for that! But believe it or not, I have heard a male medical practitioner say a very similar 'fountain of youth' thing at a recent conference here in London. He said 'any women who doesn't want to grow old early should be on HRT'.)

Wilson did assure the male readers though that their attractive and sexually active wives would not run off with another man because 'an estrogen-rich woman capable of being physically and emotionally fulfilled by her husband' was therefore unlikely to roam – unlike men, of course, for whom it was natural to have affairs, in his opinion. In fact, their marriage and even their wife's life could be saved by hormone therapy, he added, recounting the story of the Brooklyn mobster who came to see him complaining that his wife wouldn't cook anymore, she was always picking on him and was 'driving him nuts'. He produced a gun and told Wilson, 'If you don't treat her I'll kill her.' Rather than calling the police about a direct threat on a woman's life, Wilson took her as a patient and reported that: 'Her disposition improved noticeably after three weeks and soon she was very busy taking care of her sick husband.' Hallelujah! Order was restored and all was right in the world – and MHT sales quadrupled. It turned out that Wilson, who died in 1981, had received money from a pharmaceutical company that made hormone therapies at the time for the book and subsequent speaking tours, according to his son.[15]

Cutting a long story short – midlife women have always been a 'problem'. We've been diagnosed with 'climacteric insanity' and incarcerated in mad houses, called crones and witches, burnt at the stake and been subjected to bizarre treatments ranging from vaginal injections of a lead acetate solution to leeches on our vulvas – all because no one really understood what was going on. Women did complain, but no one knew why. They were indeed Haver's 'whining women' – utterly misunderstood and misdiagnosed.

But it's only Western women whining, isn't it?

This leads to another set of misconceptions about menopause – that because certain languages don't have a word for it, it doesn't exist. This is often said of Japanese and Chinese women. It's thought that in Japan, because they call the time around menopause *kōnenki* which can be translated to mean 'time of renewal' or 'change of life', and the Chinese refer to it as the 'second spring', that all is rosy and their positive attitude sees them glide on through with barely a symptom to report. This is commonly touted as a fact by companies selling supplements or nutrition plans that claim Asian women's high consumption of soy-derived phytoestrogens is the reason why they apparently sail through (see Chapter 6). But, studies show this is not the case at all – they do indeed have symptoms, but they tend to associate them with ageing rather than the end of their periods and hormone decline. Why? Because it's not something that has been talked about until recently.

Back in the 1980s, anthropologist Margaret Lock interviewed around 150 Japanese women about their experience of menopause. She published excerpts of these interviews in her 1995 book *Encounters with Aging: Mythologies of Menopause in Japan and North America*[16] where the women from various backgrounds detailed a range of symptoms, including failing eyesight, greying hair, aching joints and shoulder pain, tiredness, depression, irritability, headaches, dizziness, loss of libido and vasomotor symptoms. She found there was no clear consensus on the meaning of the word *kōnenki*. It was instead a cluster of 'amorphous' and 'relatively unstable concepts' based on experience or their beliefs or ideas. One woman called *kōnenki* 'mother's time of rebellion' and another said she'd heard women become irritable with 'heads so heavy they can't get out of bed'. Yet another said she had hot flushes and she found them embarrassing, but they weren't such an issue for a different interviewee who said, 'I just thought it was because of my age.' One woman described how it wasn't worth complaining about her symptoms because her husband would just tell her to 'shut up'.

Only 11.4 per cent of the women reported vasomotor symptoms and none said they woke drenched in sweat in the middle of the night. Lock wrote: 'By far the majority of people gave the impression that, although there is plenty of gossip and banter about *kōnenki*, much of it negative, in general it is not a subject that generates a great deal of anxiety or concern.' But, she added, as an 'augury for the future, as a sign of an aging and weakening physical body, it is not particularly welcome'.

More recently a study looking at ethnic background and menopause symptoms in Japanese women living in Hawaii found that in comparison to American women, women of Japanese descent were less likely to report any of the 30 symptoms they were asked to report on, including hot flushes. But when they were wearing a device that recorded the number of flushes they had, there were no significant differences between the two groups. The researchers concluded cultural issues were at play: 'The common finding of fewer reported HFs [hot flushes] in people of Japanese ancestry may be a consequence of reporting bias: JAs [Japanese Americans] report fewer symptoms of many conditions compared to people from other ethnic groups. This is likely due to cultural conceptions of what is appropriate to report.'[17]

A small 2020 study of 187 Chinese women found that '83.4% of participating women experienced hot flashes and 82.9% reported night sweats, with nearly half reporting moderate to severe VMS [vasomotor symptoms] (more than 3 times per day, or rated 4 or greater on a 1–8 severity scale). The median duration for both hot flashes and night sweats was 4.5 years.'[18]

A larger study of 6,364 Chinese women found that 29 per cent had vasomotor symptoms. The other reported symptoms were mood swings (37.2 per cent), insomnia (44.7 per cent), UTIs (15 per cent), sexual problems (21 per cent), itchy skin (10.5 per cent), palpitations (21.6 per cent), headaches (36 per cent), muscle and joint pain (31.6 per cent), fatigue (40.4 per cent), dizziness (31.8 per cent) and depression (18 per cent).[19]

So, it clearly isn't true to say Japanese and Chinese women don't experience menopausal symptoms – they may be less likely for cultural reason to report them, but they do have them! (And it's the same in Korea, the Philippines, India and Taiwan – the symptoms may vary but they do have them.)[20,21] And the other thing we know is that Asian women are more likely to develop osteoporosis as they age, but they are less likely to experience a major fracture.[22]

Vikram Talaulikar says there's a very simple explanation as to why no one complained before:

> They were never allowed to voice what they were going through. There's a simple answer to that, and I can see it in my own family. Even after I became an OB/GYN or a gynae resident in India, nobody talked about menopause. I saw my mother going through menopause, and I was a gynae, and never thought of asking her about it or discussing options. It was just accepted as part of life. So, I think the problem is that there is no good research, no data collection. All these women experience menopause in the same way as western populations. Yes, there are ethnic differences, age, what type of symptoms you get will differ, and that's part of any other medical condition. Everyone will be different based on geography or ethnicity, but, it's not that it doesn't exist. It's just that it's not discussed, which is why there are no papers, there is no research data about the symptomatology, and they will probably have a similar trajectory to everyone else in the world. Hopefully we can now take this menopause revolution elsewhere, so that they start talking about it, and once they start talking about it, they will realize they're all having it, and they all be able to access these options if they need them.

Change your attitude!

The other thing that flows from this is that because Asian women call it a 'time of renewal' or 'a second spring' it's hypothesised that they have fewer symptoms (which we've already established isn't correct) because they view it positively and are held in respect in their respective societies. I'm not sure how much respect the women who said her husband would tell her to 'shut up' if she complained about her symptoms was held in, but it seems to be a simplistic argument that has its roots in 1940s and 1950s studies when, for example, Chinese families traditionally lived under one roof and shared the care of their older relatives. But a more recent study that reviewed a swathe of others shows the changes in society towards a more individualistic 'nuclear family' have meant that:

- older Chinese people are now often alone and have poorer mental health and depression

- Chinese students were more negative about older adults than their American counterparts
- younger Hong Kong residents regarded their elders as 'high in warmth but low in competence'.

The conclusion was the status of older people in China was diminishing.[23] Perhaps this explains why they are now starting to report more symptoms, as they are no longer as well supported as they were in the past.

It's argued that Western societies have focused on the negative, that the next generation are now scared to death of menopause and that because of these negative attitudes they're concerned that they're really going to go through hell. We need to reframe. And yes, to some extent we do. Menopause is not the end of life – there are plenty of amazing women doing amazing things and according to Professor Joyce Harper from University College London, who has documented the secrets of 51 menopausal women, attitude does matter but looking after yourself is the key (see Chapter 12).

Evolution

Prior to his election, US Vice President JD Vance was accused of agreeing with a comment made on a podcast by a host who contended that the sole purpose of postmenopausal women was to look after grandchildren. Snopes, a fact checking resource, says it's hard to say if he agreed with the statement of not, but either way, he got a lot of criticism for it because it sounds horrendously misogynistic.

The discussion was about the 'grandmother hypothesis', which is an attempt to answer the evolutionary mystery of why humans go through menopause (as do some types of whales and narwhals, one type of chimpanzee and, it's now said, giraffes).

It's a theory developed in the 1950s, firstly by an anthropologist called Peter Medawar who compared postmenopausal women with sterile worker bees. (Of course he did!) They help clean up, provide food for the larvae, and in general look after the queen bee and the hive. A few decades later this was expanded upon by anthropologist Kristen Hawkes who studied the Hadza hunter-gatherers in Tanzania and concluded that mothers evolved to stop reproducing because it was advantageous to them (less risky than pregnancy) and then they could help their children with food gathering and child rearing.[24] Or, to put that another way, because we live longer and look after the grandkids, our daughters have been able to produce more children, and secure the future of mankind. But the theory has its critics.

One is journalist Elizabeth Landau who wrote in the *Smithsonian*: 'It's heart-warming to think of grandmothers as evolutionary heroines, especially in the face of an alternative narrative: that postmenopausal women merely represent evolution's failure to sustain fertility throughout a woman's entire life. But to sceptics, the Grandmother Hypothesis remains a "just so" story, a tidy narrative that can't truly be proven or disproven.'[25]

Men appear to get off lightly on this one too, with critics saying it underestimated the role of men or other family members who were gathering food and supporting the family. The theory is that these older women concentrated on the children of their offspring because they knew they were direct descendants, so they weren't wasting time looking after progeny that may not be related to them (so much for the proverb 'it takes a village to raise a child') but, the critics say, they weren't alone in doing this.[26]

Another argument against it is that women were often married off and sent far away from home so the grandmother was irrelevant. But, in support of the 'grandmother hypothesis', they do appear to have a positive effect on the number of children produced by their offspring and how long they live. A study looking at church records of families living near Quebec between 1621 and 1799 showed that if the daughters remained close to home they did indeed have more children (2.08 more) than those who were sent far away, and those offspring were 1.14 times more likely to live to 15 years of age.[27]

But the grandmother theory isn't the only one in town. In 2008, Lorena Madrigal and Mauricio Meléndez-Obando delivered their theory – the 'Mother Hypothesis'. They studied the descendants of families who lived in a small village in Costa Rica between the 1500s and 1900s and concluded there was a strong argument to question the grandmother hypothesis because their data showed it was 'advantageous for women to cease reproduction and concentrate their resources and energy in raising the children already produced' rather than the next generation.[28]

Either way, postmenopausal women were clearly performing some useful role, but in today's world where mothers and grandmothers in many countries are working well into their 60s before they can even qualify for a pension (albeit one that's a lot lower than men's – see Chapter 5) neither of these theories on why we 'still exist' (as insulting as that is) may seem very relevant. So, I'm putting my friend's dermatologist's comments that we shouldn't be alive into the 'myth busted' basket.

And, the fact that these women have lived long enough to go through menopause for a good few centuries, which allowed them to be studied in the first place, conveniently leads me to the next point that is often stated: women never lived this long before, and that the only reason life expectancy has risen recently is because child mortality rates have dropped. Often said, rarely challenged, but is it true?

Our World in Data, a project that's part of the UK charity Global Change Data Lab, has done some useful number crunching that shows this argument is – and I quote – 'untrue'.[29] The author Max Roser, Professor in Global Data Analytics at Oxford University, explains: 'If this were true, this would mean that we've become much better at preventing young children from dying, but have achieved nothing to improve the survival of older children, adolescents and adults.' Instead, he says the data shows that 'life expectancy has increased at all ages. The average person can expect to live a longer life than in the past, irrespective of what age they are.'

Child mortality is the number of children who die, not just in childbirth but up to the age of 5. If you take that out of the equation the figures for England and Wales show that people who made it to 5 in 1841, for example, could expect to live to the age of 55 – some longer, some shorter – it's an average. A 5-year-old born in 2020, however, could expect to live to 82, that's 27 years longer. His data shows that the average life expectancy in England and Wales in the 1700s to mid-1800s was pretty low, between 30 and 40. But again, it's an average – some lived longer, some shorter. The other point is that while the average age of menopause is around 51 in developed countries now, and late 40s in developing countries, it may have been earlier centuries ago. Back in ancient Greece, Aristotle estimated that women went through menopause at around 40, rising to 45 in the

Middle Ages, but there are arguments about how much data there is to support this latter claim.[30]

But, again, myth busted: some women have always lived long enough to go through menopause, and life expectancy increases aren't just because less babies are dying.

You'll be OK on 'the other side'

And then there's this. I'm not going to lie – this drives me batty. Once you've 'gone through' menopause you are postmenopausal and you are this way for the rest of your life. Those hormones aren't coming back. In fact, because we're living longer, we could spend 30–50 years or so as postmenopausal women, maybe even more. So, when you've gone through it that *is* the 'other side'. Yes, the vasomotor symptoms and mood swings may subside over time, although some women will have them into their 80s or beyond, and your brain fog may lift but you've got a whole host of other issues to contend with – the vaginal and bladder symptoms that can start after menopause, weakening bones and an increased risk of fragility fractures, as well as an increased risk of heart disease, metabolic disease and dementia. Yes, you may feel more comfortable in your own skin and not care as much about what others think, and you may be ecstatic that you're no longer having periods, but – and I'm not trying to be pessimistic about it – it may not all be a bed of roses where you wake up thinking 'thank God that's over!' Some symptoms persist and some new ones may start, and there are serious health implications that you need to take into consideration (see Part 3).

Ultimately, we may argue about the purpose of menopause, but three things are clear:

- Since the day dot, those of us who've lived long enough have gone through it.
- You don't have to suffer in silence.
- We are now living much longer after menopause, which is why the silent changes that happen around it that affect our heart, brain and bones are so important.

2

WHY IT MATTERS – MISOGYNY AND MONEY

All my life I've believed that men and women have equal capacities and talents . . . consequently there should be equality in life's chances.

– Julia Gillard

4

Menopause, misogyny and the year of bleeding endlessly

If you're a bit squeamish, here's your chance to skip a few pages because this is going to get a little messy.

Let me introduce to you Dr John Rutter and his friend, J.S. I take my hat off to this lady who spent most of her adult life in excruciating pain, and wanted to ensure that what couldn't be explained in life would be in her death.

J.S. lived in Liverpool and died in 1807 at 77, a good old age for the time. According to Rutter, who wrote an account of her case for the *Edinburgh Medical and Surgical Journal*[1] a year after her death, J.S. was certain her uterus was the cause of her ills. She had asked Rutter, the executor of her estate, to ensure that upon her death there would be a thorough investigation. In accordance with her wishes he asked two of his surgeon colleagues to conduct an autopsy, paying particular attention to 'the contents of her pelvis'.

But, before we get to the details of what they found, let me run you through his account of the last 50 or so years of her life.

There was nothing remarkable about the first 27 years except that her 'constitution occasionally exhibited a disposition to hysterical affections'. But things started to go wrong after she was married. She quickly became pregnant and at 29, after a difficult, long and laborious delivery, gave birth to a stillborn child. Her misfortunes didn't end there. Post-partum J.S. developed a 'miliary infection', a name given back then to infections that caused high fever and sweats, and were often fatal.

She took nearly a year to recover from this but towards the end of that year she noticed a hard lump forming in the lower left side of her pelvis which caused her pain if she bent over. Over the next nine years or so that lump grew 'until at last it rose out of the pelvis, . . . and when it had acquired its largest bulk, appeared to the touch to be about the size of a child's head'.

(This is the point where you should really turn away if you're not into gross details.)

Eventually this giant mass ruptured, emptying its putrid, coffee-coloured contents out via her rectum. This flow went on for several months, and just when she thought it was over it would repeat itself, causing her fever and pelvic pain again and again and again.

Letters addressed to her from her doctors at the time also mentioned leucorrhea 'to an uncommon degree' – a thick whitish or greenish discharge from the vagina, which they said was the cause of her fever, back pain, nausea, weakness and fainting.

When J.S. went through menopause she complained about pain in her uterus and from the area of the previously head-sized cyst. This pain affected her 24 hours a day, interrupting her sleep. Movement made it worse, and she was anxious and depressed. She lived this way for the next 27 years – in constant pain, low mood, anxious and enduring intermittent foul-smelling discharges from her rectum.

Upon her passing, Dr Rutter's colleagues set to work diligently on their autopsy and this is what they found:

- Tumour in lower abdomen
- Gangrene of labia and anus
- Hardened faeces that had distended the colon causing it to descend into the pelvis
- The uterus was attached at the back and the top to the rectum and the intestines and 'required a considerable amount of force' to detach
- There was a cyst that exuded about two 'drachms' (approximately 50mls) of blackish bituminous liquid. The cyst ran about 2 inches down to the perineum but didn't perforate the anus.
- A hard tubercle or growth about the 'size of a raspberry' was on the uterus which was also attached to the cyst
- The uterus was small (not unexpected at 77 years of age)
- The bladder was slightly distended
- The aorta, the main artery that carries blood to the lower limbs was ossified above and below the iliac dissection, where it splits to take the blood to the legs – which may cause pelvic pain, and pain in the legs.

But because the uterus looked normal and the tubercle wasn't cancerous, the doctors concluded that 'her complaints, were all hysterical'.

Let me just recap: the woman had gangrene on her labia and anus, a frequent putrid discharge from a cyst, a uterus that was stuck to its neighbours and had to be prised off with force, a tumour, calcified poo and a distended colon, and a tubercle. What else could you conclude, except that she was making her pain up?

You may well imagine that 200 or so years later things would be different – but you'd be wrong.

In December 2024 the UK government's Women and Equalities Committee released its report into *Women's Reproductive Health Conditions*,[2] and it was damning. It highlighted a culture of medical misogyny that has left women and girls who have endometriosis, adenomyosis and heavy menstrual bleeding feeling, as they wrote, as though they have 'to "suck it up" and endure pain that interferes with every aspect of their daily lives, while their conditions worsen'.

Diagnosis is slow – on average eight years for endometriosis – and the women who gave evidence told stories of being gaslit by their doctor who told them their pain or heavy bleeding was normal.

BBC broadcaster Naga Munchetty told the committee that she had had excruciating periods that lasted 11–12 days since she was 15. They made her vomit and faint and that she was literally 'wrapped around a toilet', but she too was told this was normal. It wasn't until she was 47, a full 32 years later, that she got a diagnosis of adenomyosis, a condition where the endometrial lining grows into the muscle of the uterus. This means that every time she has a period the uterus walls swell, causing pain that can be constant and chronic.

Vicky Shattock is an endometriosis and adenomyosis campaigner who has spent most of her life in chronic pain, culminating in a hysterectomy which plunged her into surgical menopause, even though her ovaries had been left behind. This is her story:

Vicky Shattock

'I was 11 when I started my periods, they were excruciatingly heavy and painful from day one. I was 12 when I first went to my doctors with them. I was 14 when I was put on the contraceptive pill and 22 when I finally got diagnosed with endometriosis. I am 42 now and after years of suffering with endometriosis and adenomyosis, including five previous surgeries, numerous medications including hormonal treatments, fighting to be heard, fighting to be diagnosed with something other than an STD or a "water infection", fainting numerous times whilst on my period, taking days off school and work, losing a job due to taking time off for my terribly painful periods, depression and anxiety, multiple different tests and procedures, and friends, family and colleagues not understanding why I needed to pull out of plans at such short notice, I finally, on the advice of a supposed world renowned endometriosis surgeon, had a hysterectomy at the age of 35.

'My ovaries remained but my uterus, cervix and fallopian tubes were removed, and so, I naively believed, had endometriosis and years of suffering. Despite not having children, I truly believed my future was going to be so different and I could finally enjoy a pain-free life. I was so wrong, and after a lot of grief, I finally realise it was not my fault to be given such false hope.

'Despite my ovaries remaining, and being assured throughout a five minute consultation with my consultant prior to my hysterectomy, I soon shot into surgical menopause – of course I would, the blood supply to my ovaries had been cut off. No one put two and two together and thought that the awful symptoms I was getting could be down to the menopause. I was severely depressed. I was suicidal. My anxiety was through the roof, I gained a ton of weight, my hair and nails were brittle, I had terrible eczema under my eyes, and insomnia. My whole life had turned upside down and I wished for my periods to return. I would take the crippling period pain over this dark hole I was in.

'My pain was still out of control, I was in so much pain every single day, it was getting worse but no one listened or cared. In the end I required further surgery for the extensive endometriosis and it has taken until the end of last year to get my dose and type of HRT correct, but I am still in a lot of pain, possibly due to nerve damage after years of living with endometriosis, and rushed surgery during my hysterectomy.

'I am still fighting to be heard, to be believed that my pain is so bad it is affecting every single part of my life. The health profession (other than my wonderful female GP), the ones who are supposed to care, don't. I have been dismissed and pushed aside as I am just one of the millions of women who undergo a hysterectomy, which surprisingly doesn't do anything for our pain.

'In fact, it just causes more problems, problems that are not listened to or treated properly – that's the problem with misogyny in the healthcare field though: women are treated appallingly, consistently dismissed, ignored, mistreated, delayed diagnoses and I sadly can't see this ending unless we all take a stand and fight for women's health and for us to be heard.'

The most recent reply Vicky received from a specialist she'd seen about her continued pain said there wasn't much else that could be done, but noted 'she lives with her partner and two cats'. (I'm not going to say a word! Well, actually I am. This basically implies: living with pain is OK if you've got someone at home, she's a crazy cat lady, she's making it up – or both, and I'm not sure any of these are relevant.)

Endometriosis and adenomyosis aren't the only times where women's reproductive pain is dismissed and suboptimal. In 2024, Diane Danzebrink's Menopause Support conducted an online survey of women who had had hysterectomies, possibly due to those conditions, that included the removal of their ovaries – a bilateral oophorectomy. As mentioned previously, if you have your ovaries removed you are plunged into menopause. There's no slow creep of symptoms – it's pretty much 'boom, hello', and the effects on physical and mental health can be considerable. It is recommended that all those who go through early menopause due to surgical, medical or chemical reasons or POI are given hormone therapy until the average age of menopause (around 51) as the lack of it can mean they are more likely to develop osteoporosis (brittle bones), heart disease, and die early from heart disease, and neurocognitive impairment including dementia and parkinsonism.[3]

But her report, *No Ovaries, No Care*, demonstrates that this clearly is not happening and women are not being fully informed prior to surgery or after surgery, and there is a serious lack of follow-up.

Some 521 women answered the survey which showed:

- 74.5 per cent said they were not made fully aware of the potential effects of having both of ovaries removed prior to surgery
- 62.4 per cent said MHT (where appropriate) was not discussed prior to surgery
- 64.1 per cent said MHT (where appropriate) was not prescribed at time of surgery
- 39.7 per cent said they were not seen for a follow-up hospital appointment
- 63.5 per cent said they were not advised to see a GP when discharged

- 83.5 per cent said their GP was not knowledgeable enough to provide care and support for surgical menopause
- 77.2 per cent said their GP did not refer them to a menopause specialist
- 42.2 per cent said they have never been able to get the right support via the NHS
- 47.2 per cent say they had no choice but to seek private care.

Almost one-third (28 per cent) spent more than £1,000 on private care with 3.3 per cent spending more than £5,000 and 2.5 per cent spending upwards of £10,000.

This is how some of the women described their experience. One said:

'I feel completely betrayed. The gynaecologist was quick to take away my ovaries but I've now been left with low levels of oestrogen and the GP will not prescribe what I need. There's no menopause specialist in Gloucestershire. I've been left to get on with it and am now at risk of long-term problems due to these low levels.'

Another said:

'I have spent the last 13 years feeling completely alone, embarrassed and completely clueless as to what was happening to me post-surgery. I honestly thought I had early onset of dementia and have seen multiple specialists for many mystery issues that have never been solved but with hindsight all seem to be menopause related. Being so young I had no one to ask for advice from as my mum hadn't even started the menopause at that point. Incredibly empty and alone.'

And another said:

'[I] was basically told by my surgeon that I had to put up with the symptoms. No aftercare advice given at all or advice about the symptoms I would expect and only have a phone check in once a year by a nurse. GP offered antidepressants. Have now requested to see a menopause specialist but my NHS appointment keeps being cancelled.'

One woman described how she had been waiting for 19 months for an appointment while another said: 'Never been offered support or referral for surgical menopause since I had my hysterectomy at 28. I am now 31 with severe vaginal atrophy. That was never spoken about.'

Feeling alone, abandoned and starved of information, 30 per cent of these women said they'd turned to online support groups to find what they needed, while another 30 per cent said social media was their source. Now, you would hope that the Royal College of Obstetricians and Gynaecologists would step up here with a handy patient fact sheet or at least an easily findable set of guidelines, but as of January 2025 if you entered the search term 'surgical menopause' on their website there was nothing there for patients that directly addressed this. And even if you were a clinician you'd have to spend a bit of time wading back to 2021 to find a clinical guidance document on risk-reducing in salpingo-oophorectomies. The Women's Health Concern, the consumer arm of the British Menopause Society, does slightly better with a short fact sheet called 'Induced menopause in endometriosis – for patients'. In both cases, the titles of the documents don't mention the phrase 'surgical menopause' which means that many women may not know that those documents are relevant to them. But beyond that, if you aren't told you're going to be plunged into menopause, surgical or otherwise, and don't know what the symptoms of menopause are, you aren't going to Google 'induced menopause' to find the information you need.

Other areas where pain is routinely dismissed, which often affects women around menopause, is the insertion of intra uterine devices or systems (IUDs or IUSs) and hysteroscopy, particularly where a biopsy is involved. A hysteroscopy is a procedure where a rod-shaped tube is passed through the cervix with a little camera that allows doctors to have a good look at the walls, or endometrial lining, of the womb. It's often done if there is unexplained bleeding between periods or heavy bleeding, especially postmenopause, to see if there are any polyps or fibroids and remove them. Sometimes a biopsy is taken – a small sample of tissue – that is sent away to check for abnormal or potentially cancerous cells. It may also be done to remove (and replace if requested) an IUD/IUS if the threads that extend into the vagina through the cervix that are usually used to remove them have disappeared. An IUD is a device that can be used for contraception, and an IUS can be used as the progestin element of MHT to protect the endometrium, and to help control heavy or unexplained bleeding, and also to help with endometriosis.

The NHS acknowledges that this can be 'uncomfortable and may feel like period pain' and suggests that 'taking ibuprofen or paracetamol 1 hour before the procedure can help'. It also says: 'It may be possible to have a general anaesthetic or an injection to help you relax (intravenous sedation) during the hysteroscopy. Not all hospitals or clinics offer this, so you may need to be referred to one that does.'[4]

This brings me to 'the year (or more) of bleeding endlessly'. I had an IUS, a Mirena coil inserted about seven years ago. Its role in postmenopausal wombs is to protect the endometrial lining by 'opposing' the effect of the oestrogen component of MHT. Oestrogen makes the lining thick and, to steal a phrase from menopause GP Carys Sonnenberg, the progestin in the coil 'acts like a lawnmower' and stops it thickening and in turn increasing the risk of developing endometrial cancer. I know some people find having it inserted horrendous, but luckily for me, it wasn't that bad – a deep breath in, twinge and a couple of weeks of the odd cramp afterwards which felt a bit like period pain, and a little bit of spotting. For the next five years it was 'set and forget' and I had no issues. It was perfect. After five years though its use-by date was up and it needed to be replaced, and this is where it all started to go messily wrong. Having it out wasn't a problem, another deep breath, twinge, and it was over and done with, but I was told I couldn't have it replaced because NHS sexual health clinics were only funded to insert it for contraception purposes and my GP wasn't qualified to do it. Instead I was prescribed an oral progesterone tablet and this did not agree with me. Apart from the non-stop heavy bleeding, it made me (more) irritable and moody and also gave me gastric reflux – something I'd never had before. (Progesterone can cause the sphincter at the top of the stomach to relax, resulting in reflux. Who knew?) I tried to use it vaginally but it still didn't stop the bleeding, even when the dose was doubled.

When the bleeding started I was actually chairing a debate at a menopause conference and I remember standing at the podium and feeling something I hadn't felt for about a decade – an unexpected trickle that soon became a gush of blood heading for my socks. When I got off stage I scanned the room for people who looked like they were still young enough to be menstruating and bailed them up against columns and walls to fleece them of their sanitary products. I have never gone through so many, so fast, in one day. It was not pleasant. I spoke to my

GP afterwards and was told to give it six months to allow for the progesterone to kick in and do its job. It didn't so I went back, by now close to anaemic, and said 'we need to fix this'. I was referred for an ultrasound scan and there was nothing particularly untoward, so I soldiered on. A few months later the bleeding still hadn't stopped so I went for another scan and it was decided that I should indeed have another Mirena coil as the endometrium was slightly thicker than they'd like, so off I went to the hospital to have it inserted. I was told I would be having a hysteroscopy to swap them over but was not told I would be having a biopsy. I'd had a hysteroscopy before and it wasn't fun, but it wasn't too bad, but not fun – but this time it was very different. I took my ibuprofen before the procedure and they did give me a local anaesthetic in the cervix (which stung for a second or two) but that didn't cover the inside of the uterus and the area where they took the biopsy.

Over the years I've had a lot of moles, basal cell carcinoma and squamous cell carcinomas removed from my skin (thanks to a misspent youth under the Australian sun) and they always do that with a local anaesthetic. I've had what's called 'punch biopsies' too that involve taking a very small sample of skin, and these too are done with local anaesthetic – but this biopsy was not. I remember doing an audible intake of breath and may have let loose with the odd expletive for two. It wasn't the worst pain I've even endured but it really wasn't the least. I walked home and had to stop a few times due to the cramps and pain.

For the next few weeks the pain, especially on the lower left side of my abdomen, continued, as did the bleeding. I waited for it to settle. It didn't. So after about six months or so I went back to the GP and another scan was done. It showed that the coil had gone walkabout in my uterus and one arm of its T-shape couldn't be seen. We decided it should be replaced. I was referred to see a gynaecologist at the local menopause clinic who really didn't think that the ongoing bleeding or pain on one side was an issue. 'We see serious things here, like cancer,' she said. This was a menopause clinic that I'd been referred to, but OK. I explained that I was worried that the IUS may have implanted itself into the uterus wall and that may be causing the pain. She told me it was 'vary rare' and even if it were, it wasn't really an issue, it would still do its job protecting the endometrium. But if I really wanted it changed she could do it there and then along with another biopsy. I explained that I was now quite anxious about the procedure due to the previous experience and would prefer if it were done under some kind of sedation. She rolled her eyes – I do not jest – and stonily said that she'd refer me back to the original hospital.

How did I feel? Guilty, because, obviously, I was wasting people's time when there were people with more important problems to see. Embarrassed, because I was obviously a wimp, and frankly gaslit, because my pain and concerns were dismissed.

Eventually someone rang me to make an appointment for the replacement which saw me apologising over the phone about my request for pain relief because, clearly, I must be a princess. Finally, the date came and it was removed, replaced, and a biopsy done all under a general anaesthetic. Afterwards the doctor came to talk to me and showed me a picture of the coil which was indeed firmly implanted in the left side of my uterus.

I am not saying this to put anyone off having a Mirena coil because when it's good, it's very, very good and what happened to me is in fact quite rare – 1 in 1,000.[5] I included this to highlight that even gnarly people like me (not a wilting flower) get gaslit.

My experience, however, doesn't seem to be an isolated event. The Campaign Against Painful Hysteroscopy is a UK-based group that's done a survey of around 8,000 women's hysteroscopy experiences and the comments respondents made show an uncaring environment where pain is dismissed or ignored.[6] It also shows how the NHS wording may understate the extent of the pain some people experience.

Regarding the nurses in the room one woman wrote:

> She was jolly and chatty but as the procedure continued was more focussed on the consultant, and when I started going into shock, [she] started shouting at me to stop shaking and hold still. It was only when my husband noticed I was going blue that they stopped. I don't know if she would have actually noticed.

Another said:

> They wouldn't listen to the carer I had taken with me when she expressed she could clearly see me in distress. They continued on although I could feel my heart beating so fast. I was sweating and I couldn't see. I was trying so hard to focus on breathing I couldn't physically speak.

And another:

> I cried because it hurt and she told me to stop being silly and that it didn't hurt.

And another:

> I felt intimidated, there was a nurse on either side of me they seemed to hold each arm down and kept telling me it was nearly done.

And another:

> It took 2 days [for me] to fully understand that I'd passed out and then 2 weeks to get over the fact that they carried on regardless and acted as if nothing had happened.

And another:

> The shock, the way it was handled was appalling. I felt I was being attacked. This was the worst treatment I have ever experienced in my entire life not to mention humiliating and distressing, degrading, excruciating.

I could go on but I'll stop with this one:

> I walked out of the room sobbing only to see a full waiting room with 'everyone' looking shocked at me. One lady was even crying looking at me. I am left traumatised from this terrible experience. I do not think I'll ever recover.

It's possible some will be angry with me for talking about the pain and argue that it will put women off having these lifesaving – and they are lifesaving – investigations. But the point is – offer people appropriate pain relief. You wouldn't stick a camera up someone's bottom or a man's penis without appropriate pain relief – why should this be any different? Saying 'most people' get by without pain relief disregards those who don't, and expecting people to 'suck it and see' as an experiment is just asking for trouble – the damage is done. I know it costs money and these are not small numbers of people. Some 71,000 had these procedures done in 2019–20 in England alone,[7] but if you want them to come back next time should they need to, treat their pain appropriately the first time and make the options clear, or they won't.

When a 2023 government review on 'NHS Hysteroscopy Treatment' looked at who was following guidelines of offering pain management it found it was impossible to tell which clinics were.[8] In my case, for the first two hysteroscopies, simply being told to take a Panadol an hour before was not giving me the full set of options needed for an informed consent.

The difficulty in accessing pain relief, either IV sedation or a general anaesthetic, stems from the fact that services are limited because not all NHS facilities are set up to offer them. But with demand for the procedures rising, mostly among postmenopausal women due to oral progesterone not being quite as effective as everyone had hoped in preventing unexplained/unscheduled bleeding, more attention will need to be paid to address this as the number of discontented or fearful women will grow too.

It's a similar situation when it comes to getting smear tests for cervical cancer. Vaginal dryness and changes to the vaginal canal around menopause can make having a smear a living hell for many women. I cannot tell you how many times I've had women tell me that it's too painful, that they've had to ask them to stop, that they've been told it's their fault, or that they can't have lube to make it easier, which is not correct.

Blaming the patient is something Dr Shilpa McQuillan, community gynaecologist and clinical lead of the Berkshire Menopause Clinic, takes umbrage at. Having recently been a patient herself, she experienced first-hand how patients are blamed, for example when staff are unable to place cannulas into veins. This made her reflect on her own female patients, and, sadly, how women's own anatomy is often blamed for the inability to carry out a cervical screening or speculum examination. But Dr McQuillan wants us to know it's not our fault. 'Everyone is unique and we all have normal variants of anatomy.'

According to guidance from Public Health England in 2017, the number of older women attending cervical screening appointments was at a 17-year low. In England, they said, 81.6 per cent of 50–54-year-olds attended screening in 2014–15, but that dropped to

74.8 per cent of 55–59-year-olds, and 73.2 per cent of 60–64-year-olds. That's an average of 78.5 per cent of 50–64-year-olds. By 2023 that average had dropped to 74.4 per cent.[9]

Public Health England said there were two things at play here: 'A lack of knowledge about the cause of cervical cancer and who can be affected appear to be contributing to older women not attending cervical screening.' It also cited a survey by Jo's Cervical Cancer Trust which found that a third of women over 50 said the smear had become more painful with age, including a quarter who said the pain started after they went through menopause.[10]

Dr McQuillan says there are some simple steps that can avoid pain being an issue. 'In most cases, there are lots of techniques your clinician can use to make the procedure more comfortable for you. For example, if you have vulval or vaginal dryness, we can prescribe topical oestrogen for a few months leading up to the procedure; use lots of lubricant; and use a small speculum.' She says there are things you can do too to feel more at ease and empowered. 'If you feel in control, you'll be more relaxed, and this could make the procedure more comfortable – so bring music, or a friend with a hand to hold.'

The aforementioned *Women's Reproductive Health Conditions* report found: 'A common theme in the evidence received was that of women's pain being dismissed, not just due to a lack of understanding as to what might be causing it but because of a lack of empathy and "medical misogyny". Women reported not feeling listened to and being "gaslit", especially when accessing NHS services about a gynaecological issue that included pain.'[11] It cites a survey of more than 5,000 UK adults by manufacturer of the pain-reliever Nurofen, which found that 62 per cent of women that year said their pain had been ignored or dismissed by healthcare professionals, up from 49 per cent in the previous year. Some 17 per cent said their doctor had described them as 'overly dramatic' or 'emotional'.

And, when it comes to getting your doctor to take your menopause symptoms seriously, it's a similar picture. When calls were made for submissions to the *Women's Health Strategy* which came out in 2022, menopause was the third most requested topic for inclusion with 48 per cent of respondents selecting it. It cited a public survey that showed that 36 per cent of respondents felt uncomfortable talking to healthcare professionals about menopause.[12]

A 2022 Fawcett Society survey on more than 4,000 women found that 45 per cent of women hadn't spoken to their doctor about their symptoms. Of those who had, around a third (31 per cent) said it took many appointments before their GP realised they were experiencing menopause or perimenopause. Official guidance says that MHT should be offered to women who are struggling with menopause symptoms, but just 39 per cent of women said their GP or nurse offered it as soon as they knew they were experiencing symptoms, and only 14 per cent of menopausal women said that they are currently taking it. White women were almost twice as likely to be prescribed MHT than Black women or women from other minority groups.[13]

Again, the comments made to various All-Party Parliamentary Groups,[14] and the 'Women's Health – Let's talk about it' survey of some 97,000 women,[15] and those made across social media, bear a remarkable similarity with women repeatedly saying they were offered antidepressants and not hormone therapy, or were dismissed, or felt like they weren't listened to. In fact, in the 40–79 age group around 80 per cent of respondents said they felt their doctor hadn't listened to them.[16]

A 2024 survey of 1,500 women by Mumsnet found that 40 per cent didn't trust their doctor to manage their menopause, with 39 per cent of those who sought help for perimenopause symptoms and 27 per cent for menopause symptoms saying their GP told them they'd just have to learn to live with it.[17]

The 2023 Besins-funded study on doctor's attitudes mentioned earlier, which found they lacked confidence in prescribing MHT, also found that barriers to women seeking help included 'a lack of knowledge of the full range of symptoms, stigma, embarrassment and the belief that it is part of normal ageing. Previous negative experience in accessing advice or treatment discouraged women from pursuing help.' It said there were 'multiple opportunities to address these gaps in knowledge, including . . . education and culturally appropriate leaflets to reach a wider range of perimenopausal and menopausal women'.[18]

So, again, you'd expect that calls for a public awareness campaign would be universally supported. But again, you'd be wrong. Numerous campaign groups including Menopause Support, Menopause Mandate and the Menopause Research and Education Fund, along with the multiple reports mentioned above, have called for one, and the

Women's Health Strategy itself found that just 9 per cent of respondents said they had enough information about the menopause. But the government has rejected the call claiming it's not necessary. It says it's updated the NHS website and that it has a set of tools on the way, and that should suffice.

'There's some great information on some of these stakeholder websites. But how do you know to go and look at that information?' asks Danzebrink. 'Why would you go there, because you're not aware that that stuff exists? And I think the thing is, maybe 20 years ago people would have gone to "the internet" to a website. They might have "Googled" something but people don't do that anymore. They go to Instagram and TikTok, and if you're not there, and you're not there regularly and you're not there saying "we are the authority, and this is the factual, evidence-based information," well, people aren't going to go and look for it on a website.'

This is especially poignant if you remember the statistic that 9 per cent of women felt they had enough information about menopause. If they don't know what the symptoms of menopause are they aren't going to search for menopause, let alone visit a website because they don't know what they've 'got', for want of a better word. So, we're in a classic catch-22 situation.

The NHS website attracts around 40 million clicks per month, but it's impossible to say how many are looking at the menopause pages. I did a quick analysis of 'traffic', that is the number of people who visit websites, on other sites that deliver menopause information for the public. In November 2024 the UK's 'Rock My Menopause' site, which draws information from the Primary Care Women's Health Forum that provides education and resources for medical practitioners, attracted just under 5,000 visitors that month. The Women's Health Concern received about 29,000 visitors, and a site set up in the US called 'My Meno Plan', which is government-funded but run by healthcare professionals, attracted – wait for it – a whopping 2,500 visitors. Bear in mind it's estimated that 6,000 women enter menopause every day in the US[19] and there are around 13 million perimenopausal or menopausal women in the UK[20] and by 2030 there are expected to be 1.2 billion globally.[21] So, you'd expect a lot more traffic than this on 'official' sites.

You would also expect sites like 'Newson Health' with Dr Louise Newson's 700,000-plus Instagram following to get a huge amount of traffic but even her site only attracted 15,000. Another popular figure on Instagram is US-based Dr Jen Gunter, an author, obstetrician and gynaecologist who is known for taking those she doesn't think are adhering to the evidence, to task. She has around 300,000 followers and her website had around 30,000 visitors. The exception was Mary Claire Haver, with around 7 million followers on various platforms at the time of writing, who attracted 257,000 or so website visitors, but she does have a shop on her site selling supplements – so they may not have been there for the menopause content alone. (If you're into tech – the bounce rate varied from around 41 per cent to 63 per cent – that's a measure of how long some stays on a page. If someone lands on a page and spends less than a couple of seconds they've 'bounced' and the content wasn't for them. The highest bounce rates were on the Women's Health Concern and Jen Gunter's sites, and the lowest was on 'Rock My Menopause' and Mary Claire Haver's sites. The amount of time spent on these sites ranged from 0.43 seconds to just under 6 minutes (Women's Health Concern and Rock My Menopause topped those). The number of pages looked at ranged from 1.67 to 3.15 and the average was 2.4. Again, those last two sites scored best – so when people want quality info, they'll stay and read, but the number is nothing in comparison to the hits on social media.

I randomly picked ten of Mary Claire Haver's posts and the average number of people who viewed them was 475,000. For Dr Jen Gunter it was 180,000, for Dr Louise Newson it was 83,000 – and my point from all those stats is that: yes, you must have a website, but seriously, that's not where people are finding their information.

'You can't expect people to find information on something that they know nothing about. You need to bring it to them. And it's the same with things like NICE guidance and British Menopause Society guidelines. You have to bring those things to the people. You can't expect them to go and find them. They're way behind the curve on this,' Danzebrink says.

She'd like to see a televised campaign, posters on buses, in pubs, on toilet doors in workplaces – anywhere where women are, but in the UK at the moment that seems highly unlikely (see Chapter 11).

5

Sex, drugs and the menoconomy

It's a sad fact that in order to get menopause, or women's health in general, taken seriously it has to be presented as an economic argument. Fortunately, there are a number of reports that show just how much menopause costs the economy and why investing in women's health, including menopause, can give it a significant boost.

One of these is a January 2024 report from the McKinsey Health Institute called *Closing the Women's Health Gap: A $1 Trillion Opportunity to Improve Lives and Economies*.[1] As its name suggests, the report argues that investing in women's health, including menopause, could add $1 trillion to the global economy by 2040.

How? By supporting women as they hit menopause, and by increasing our 'health span'. You're probably well acquainted with the term 'life span' but let me introduce you to the term 'health span' in case you're not so familiar with that one. Life span refers to our longevity or how many years we live. Health span, on the other hand, refers to how many years we spend in good health. And for women, the news isn't good.

The way the researchers measure health span is by looking at what's called DALYs, or disability adjusted life years. This is a measure of the burden of disease which, according to the World Health Organization (WHO), takes into account premature mortality as well as years spent in ill health or due to disability. And it turns out that although women may live a few years longer than men we spend 25 per cent more time than our male counterparts – around nine years more – in poor health, and that represents a significant blow not only to our quality of life but also to the economy. As the report says it 'affects her ability to be present and/or productive at home, in the workforce, and in the community and reduces her earning potential'.

And it's not just the earning potential, it's pensions and superannuation too. Maternity leave, childcare, caring for elderly loved ones, absences due to illness – many of which are related to reproductive health – combine to see our pension pots and superannuation considerably reduced. Add to that the number of women who cut back on working hours or retire early due to menopause and there's a significant blow to what we have left to retire on.

One actuarial report shows that lower-income earners at the start of their working lives who take two years' maternity leave and return to work three days a week after the birth of the first child 'could end up missing out on between £20,000 and £50,000 by the time they reach state pension age, depending on how many years they work part-time'.[2]

A railway workers' report called *Mind the Gender Pension Gap* puts the figures starkly showing the time we take out as unpaid 'carers' sees 'women retire with average pension savings of £69,000 compared to £205,000 for men. This gap of £136,000 worth of pension savings means that a woman would have to work an extra 19 years to be able to bridge it and to afford the same level of retirement savings as a man.'[3] That means you're retiring at around 84 – unfortunately that's a year or so longer than you're expected to live if you live in the UK, so you're literally working yourself into the grave. Figures from NOW Pensions shows that 67 per cent of the pensioners living in poverty are women, and 64 per cent of those are single women.[4]

But it's not just caring for kids, it's caring for our parents too – welcome to the sandwich generation. Not only are we simultaneously juggling tweens and teens and all those hormones in one house, we're also taking time out to care for elderly or unwell parents – and this can cost families a lot. In the UK, home care for the elderly and unwell is means tested and 2021 figures show it was not available to people with assets worth more than £23,250.[5] Even when you are eligible, there's not enough of it. For the vast majority, it's self-funded or taken on by spouses while they're well enough, or other family members. 2021 census data shows that 5.8 million people were providing unpaid care in the UK and Carer's UK reports that 1.7 million we're providing more than 50 hours a week in care. Almost two-thirds (59 per cent) were women.[6]

If a value were put on all these hours of unpaid work it would come to £184 billion a year, according to a 2024 report from the Centre for Care, published in partnership with Carers UK.[7] Just to put that into perspective, the report says: 'The combined NHS budget across the four nations of the UK in 2021/2022 was £189 billion – meaning that carers are providing the value of care equivalent to a second NHS.'

The impact?

- 2 million unpaid carers live in poverty, 400,000 are in deep poverty.
- A quarter are 'not in good health'.
- 7 million are not in paid employment.
- 6 million, or around 600 a day, have given up work.[8]

Carers UK estimates that the average loss of earnings is £12,000 per carer. Multiply that by ten years or so and add on the loss of super-annuation contributions and you've got another considerable hole in your pocket, not to mention the impact on any potential state pension.

And these loss estimates haven't even taken into account the costs of time off, retiring early or cutting back on work hours due to menopause symptoms, but there are reports that are starting to show that it is indeed having an impact. One recent report, called *The Menopause Penalty* from the Institute of Fiscal Studies, suggests the losses are substiantial. The researchers wrote: 'Our baseline estimates show that, four years after a menopause-related diagnosis, earnings decline by 10% relative to the year before diagnosis – driven by both reduced work hours and early labor market exit. These effects vary significantly: the negative impacts are concentrated among women without a college degree. Moreover, losses are most pronounced for those working in larger firms and in workplaces with a higher share of female coworkers aged 45 and older.'[9]

When it comes to the economy, we're starting to see a body of work outlining the costs. In 2023, the Mayo Clinic in the US published the results of a survey of 32,469 of its patients aged between 45 and 60.[10] Its aim was to evaluate the impact of menopause symptoms in the workplace and estimate the cost to the economy. Some 16.1 per cent, or 5,200, of those who were invited to take part responded and of those around 85 per cent, or 4,440, were employed at the time.

The researchers rated the severity of symptoms using the Menopause Rating Scale, which is one of the tools commonly used in menopause research. They found the mean score was 12.1, which they said correlated with moderate menopause symptoms, but as the severity increased, the likelihood of taking time off work increased too. The survey found that 597 of the respondents (13.4 per cent) reported at least one adverse work outcome due to menopause symptoms and

10.8 per cent, or 485, said they had missed one or more days of work in the year before the study due to their symptoms. Based on the number of days off, the researchers calculated menopause symptoms were costing the US economy $1.8 billion a year, and again that doesn't include costs that are related to reduced hours of working, changing jobs or retiring early due to menopause symptoms.

Working out how many people leave their jobs because of menopause is no easy task, and there are arguments about the robustness of some of the statistics that are commonly cited. An example of this is the figure of 900,000 women who are said to have left work in the UK because of menopause, which has been cited in numerous news articles and various government reports. The statistic comes from a small 2019 study of 1,000 women that looked at a variety of events that affect women including pregnancy, fertility, periods and menopause.[11] It was commissioned by BUPA and conducted by Censuswide and found that 4 per cent of women had left work due to symptoms for all of these, not just menopause. This 4 per cent was later extrapolated to the entire female working-age population of around 22 million to deliver the figure of 900,000 women walking out the door, and that was then attributed to their menopause symptoms. So based on that study it's not entirely correct to say just under a million women have quit because of menopause. With around 5 million menopausal women in the workforce, depending on whose figures you look at, it would be closer to 200,000. (Credit here to Magnificent Midlife who questioned the figure first and traced it back to its source.[12]) But there are many other surveys showing similar results, so there's definitely a trend that's hard to deny. One of those is the Fawcett Society report *Menopause and the Workplace*, which surveyed 4,014 women between the ages of 40 and 55 and found that 1 in 10 women who had worked during menopause had left their job due to their symptoms.[13]

A British Medical Association survey of 2,000 female healthcare workers is particularly disturbing as the UK's national health provider, the NHS, in 2024 had about 30,000 female workers aged 45–55.[14]

It found:

- 93 per cent of survey respondents had experienced menopause symptoms
- 90 per cent said that these had impacted their working lives
- 38 per cent said the impact was significant
- 36 per cent had made changes to their working lives as a result of menopause (such as reducing working hours or changing jobs)
- 38 per cent wanted to make changes to their working lives as a result of menopause but said they couldn't
- 16 per cent had discussed their menopause symptoms with their manager
- 47 per cent wanted to discuss it but did not feel comfortable doing so.

Sexist and ageist behaviour among management were cited as reasons for not discussing the symptoms, with women fearing it would damage their career progression.

The authors wrote that there was 'a concerning number of respondents who said they had or intended to leave medicine early. A clear theme throughout these kinds of responses is that they still enjoyed their career but found they just couldn't manage their symptoms at work. As one doctor said, "I left a job I loved."'

CIPD, the Chartered Institute of Personnel and Development, released a report too based on a survey of 2,000 women aged 40–60 in the UK, which found that 17 per cent had considered leaving their jobs and a further 6 per cent had. It also found that more than 10 per cent of women felt discriminated against as a result of their menopause symptoms.[15] Another survey by workplace healthcare provider, Simply Health, found 23 per cent of the 2,000 women it surveyed had considered resigning while 14 per cent said they were going to quit.[16] Madhu is one of those who did. This is her story.

On 1 February 2016 Madhu woke up and told her husband, 'I'm going to resign today' after more than 20 years as recruitment specialist with a government organisation.

In her early 40s, Madhu noticed changes in her nails and hair. Her periods were still regular and the GP did blood tests and found she had no deficiencies. Her children were now almost independent and she was starting to spend more time with her husband. Life was generally good. She was an independent worker who loved her job, had no difficulties attending and presenting at meetings and had formed good relationships with the internal and external groups she worked with. But things began to change.

'I thought my 40s was going to be my time where I could work on myself and my career; however, there had been a number of management changes in a few short years and at that time, I think, I started changing, feeling withdrawn.

'I wasn't able to sleep and I had migraines every week for a day or two days, and I'd have a few days after that where I felt absolutely drained. And the night sweats. I was completely drenched. I'd have to get up, and then at 2.30 in the morning I'd be wide awake. And being wide awake meant that I wasn't sleeping. This would also be the time when I would worry constantly about the smallest things and start panicking. I still had no knowledge about what was happening to me. But then when the periods were becoming irregular I would miss a month, then bleed twice a month, it would be very, very heavy. And I think for me, because I never had issues with my periods, that became an issue. I wasn't used to that. Then I was regularly going to the GP and they did do a blood test because I was under 45 to check to if it was the start of the menopause or anything, but the results would always come back negative. So, I had no conversation and was referred to a gynaecologist. The gynaecologist never mentioned anything about perimenopause. All he actually said was that "it's the hormones". But that, to me, doesn't mean it's the perimenopause or it's the menopause. I didn't even know what perimenopause meant.

'I just dealt with it and coped with it. The sleepless nights and night sweats were an issue because it was every single night. And you know, as a woman, we're still expected to be that same individual, and you just carry on and be the same person that I was at work and at home. Emotionally, though, I was drained. I was impacted. I needed reassurance from my employer that I was doing my job well when I was never like that before. And then the uncertainty began, and I just didn't feel right.

'I was just going to work for the sake of work now, not the fact that I liked it. And I just didn't know what was happening to me. And I had no answers. The GP wasn't giving me an answer. And I was just left to my own devices to carry on, and that's what I was trying to do. But my mind was going insane, crazy. I wasn't coping, and my marriage was breaking down, and the way I thought about my husband started changing.

I didn't feel right within myself. In my mind, I was definitely distanced and just wasn't happy. And I think my girls felt it, and they felt the environment in the house, they didn't know what to expect every day when they came home. I felt alone. I started to get depressed, I didn't value myself. I felt I wasn't giving anything and I wasn't bringing anything home. I had changed from being this independent, confident individual to just wanting to be indoors and not meet anyone and not see anyone. My confidence had completely gone. I was completely withdrawn. I couldn't make decisions. I just changed completely, and I didn't like the person that I had become. But alongside that, I would get angry with the family because when it comes to us as women, we just try and carry on and we suffer in silence, but are still there for everyone which means we're actually at the bottom of the list. And I would get angry with my family, thinking that they should know that I need help, but I wasn't talking about the fact that I needed help. So, they didn't. They didn't know what was happening. My husband didn't know what was happening and our relationship was crumbling. The whole life was crumbling.'

Madhu had been tearful and vulnerable at work. After an incident where she felt she had been picked on and embarrassed in a meeting, she built up the courage to talk to her manager about her symptoms but instead of finding an empathetic ear the only thing the manager was concerned about was if she would be able to meet her targets.

A few months later, when she woke that February morning she thought to herself, *there's only 28 days in the month*, and turned to her husband to say, 'I'm going to resign today.' She recalls, 'It just came out of nowhere, and I was so relieved.'

Her eldest daughter stepped in and told her she needed to see someone and get some help. Her previous GP had told her to take Black Cohosh and wouldn't prescribe MHT. But she took the opportunity to see a locum who did prescribe it and after doing some research she realised that she had around 50 per cent of the 30 or so symptoms usually ascribed to menopause. MHT wasn't a 'miracle pill' but it was a 'life-saver', she says. Now, she says she's 'back. Back, with a bit of a voice on me.'

Madhu now works to support women and raise awareness in workplaces about menopause – and she's loving it.

Clearly, Madhu isn't alone, and even if the studies vary in the size of the problem, they all paint a picture of brain drain and economic loss that can't be ignored if you want a fully functioning economy.

It's a point that was picked up by the NHS Confederation in its October 2024 report *Women's Health Economics: Investing in the 51 Per Cent*.[17] It looked at menstrual dysfunction (heavy bleeding, period pain, endometriosis), perimenopause (which often sees exacerbated symptoms), menopause and mental health, and found there was a considerable cost to the UK economy.

Using Office of National Statistics data on absenteeism and presenteeism (turning up but not functioning properly) it drew several conclusions. For period pain:

- Women with severe period pain miss 18 days of work per year due to their symptoms.
- Women with heavy periods miss 11 days of work per year due to their symptoms.
- Women with secondary dysmenorrhea (painful periods caused by an underlying condition like endometriosis) miss 16 days of work per year due to their symptoms.
- 30 per cent of those experiencing endometriosis take more than three days off per month due to period pain, compared to 6 per cent of those who do not experience endometriosis.

The cost of absenteeism:

- due to severe pain during periods: £3.7 billion per year
- due to heavy periods: £4.7 billion per year
- due to secondary dysmenorrhea: £2.2 billion per year

The cost of presenteeism:

- due to severe pain during periods: £291.9 million per year
- due to heavy periods: £418.1 million per year
- due to secondary dysmenorrhea: £173.0 million per year

When it came to perimenopause and menopause, the report looked at a narrow window of women aged 45–55 and the impact of the following eight symptoms: difficulty sleeping, low mood or anxiety, hot flushes, night sweats, vaginal dryness, discomfort during sex, reduced sex drive and problems with memory or concentration.

It found that those with all eight symptoms were less likely to be in employment than the rest of the population (83 per cent versus

89 per cent respectively). Like the BMA, it cited women saying they felt 'isolated and lonely'.

Those with all eight symptoms were also 20 per cent more likely to take time off each month. Of those who didn't take time off, 76 per cent said they wanted to. As one woman put it: 'The only reason I don't take sick days is because I work from home. If I didn't, I would have to take about six months a year off.'

They concluded that there were around 60,000 women not in employment as a result of the perimenopause or menopause, and calculated that if they were working and earning the average wage for their age, approximately £1.5 billion could be added to the economy each year.

This, they said, was a conservative figure that didn't take into account other economic factors such as savings from 'reduced welfare payments, the indirect and induced impact associated with any increases in income (i.e. the "ripple effect" caused by individuals spending more money), or the savings employers realise in not having to hire and train new employees'.

Data presented to a parliamentary working committee by Health and Her®, a supplement manufacturer, from a 2019 survey of 1,004 women also conducted by Censuswide showed that hot flushes, memory loss, joint aches and anxiety are just some of the menopause symptoms that reportedly cost the UK economy 14 million working days every year, which equates to an approximate £1.8 billion loss to the UK economy.[18]

When it came to the way the women felt the NHS Confederation report estimated that around 370,000 menopausal women were 'miserable or depressed' and experiencing poor mental health. It also found, not surprisingly, that those with more severe symptoms were more likely to class their health as 'poor' or 'fair'. Those with eight symptoms were almost twice as likely to report that their health is 'bad' or 'very bad' compared to those experiencing one menopause symptom (11 per cent compared to 6 per cent). Supporting these women makes sense, it says. For every additional £1 spent in obstetrics and gynaecology services per woman in England, there would be an estimated return on investment of £11 and an additional £319 million would be added to the economy.

But it's not just how we feel and cope when we go through peri- to postmenopause that matters. It's the silent changes that rob us of our health span later on, and these cost the economy dearly too.

Heart disease for both genders costs the UK health system £7.4 billion, with an annual cost to the wider economy of £15.8 billion[19] and remember – heart disease is one of the biggest killers of women and our risk of having a heart attack matches men's by around the age of 65. In the US, the *Women's Health and Health Care Reform: The Economic Burden of Disease* report[20] looked at diseases in women and the costs in 2009 and found that the annual direct costs of various diseases were indeed considerable. It found the direct costs of the following:

- cardiovascular disease, which affects 43 million American women, was approximately $162 billion
- depression was estimated to be over $20 billion
- osteoporosis, which affects nearly 8 million American women, was nearly $14 billion
- diabetes was over $58 billion
- breast cancer was around $9.1 billion.

It said the 'Centers for Medicare and Medicaid Services (CMS), which pays a portion of these direct medical costs for women over 65 and disabled women, reports that for women alone it will spend $33.7 billion for cardiovascular disease, $4.4 billion for depression, $4.8 billion for diabetes, and over $0.8 billion for mammography in FY 2009'.

These are not small sums, and with an ageing population aren't likely to go down unless there is a substantial investment in women's health and research to see why some postmenopausal women are more vulnerable to these conditions than others, and what treatments work best (see Part 3).

These unfortunately aren't the only conditions that affect women. We are more likely to suffer from immune diseases, back pain, headaches, musculoskeletal disorders, Alzheimer's disease and other types of dementia, as well as depressive disorders and anxiety, according to the *Global Burden of Disease* report.[21] And when it comes to what kills us, depending on which country you live in, there are a few conditions that regularly appear in the top five and they include heart disease (as we mentioned), strokes, dementia and Alzheimer's.

So, it's not surprising that the McKinsey report targets cardiovascular and cerebrovascular disease as a major priority to tackle. It singles out a particular type called ischaemic heart disease (where the blood flow is blocked to part of the heart) and stroke as major contributors to the global burden of disease accounting for 16 per cent of DALYs for men and 14 per cent for women. When women have heart attacks the signs and symptoms are often unrecognised and as a result we are less likely to be referred to for diagnostic or interventional procedures in comparison to men.[22] And if we are referred and have a stent, a common treatment for opening up blocked arteries to improve blood flow to the heart muscle, we are more likely to die afterwards than our male counterparts[23] (see Chapter 8).

The solution, it says, is to invest in health research. It says the return on investment for every $1 spent in high-income countries on research will be $3.50 and around $2.00 in lower-income countries.

But to date there hasn't been much of an appetite for research that involves women. Up until 1993 in the US it wasn't mandatory at all to include women in research and as a result we now have what's called a 'data gap' – a huge hole in our knowledge when it comes to medications for common conditions that affect both sexes. Because of that we have two significant problems – we don't really know how well certain drugs work in women, and women are more likely to suffer from adverse effects from the medications they take in comparison to men.

One *Lancet* report found there were around 9 million adverse effects reported by women on the WHO's VigiBase, a global databank of individual case safety reports, in comparison to 6 million or so by men between 1967 and 2018.[24] Another study showed women were 50–75 per cent more likely to have an adverse reaction to a drug than their male counterparts.[25] And FDA data shows that women were 36 per cent more likely to have a serious adverse reaction or to die from an adverse reaction than men, with 8.3 million reports involving women recorded compared to 6.1 million for men from 2000–22, the McKinsey report says.

There are a number of theories relating to why this happens including that:

- dosages are based on male studies but women are generally much smaller so they're taking too much
- women may metabolise drugs differently
- women are more likely to take more medications than men and therefore have a higher rate of adverse reactions.

This last point is a proposition put forward by Harvard researchers, who postulate that social and environmental factors such as poverty and violence, which are associated with higher rates of chronic illness and mental health problems, conspire to see women consuming more medications. They argue that if you take these factors into account the real disparity in female versus male over-reporting drops to around 5 per cent.[26] (Although why we need to take those into account is another question altogether, because – utopian thought, I know – they shouldn't be there in the first place.)

Traditionally women were excluded from clinical trials for a number of sometimes contradictory reasons:

- 'bikini medicine' – the belief that women really weren't that different from men except for having bigger boobs and no penis
- our annoying fluctuating hormones that could interfere with results
- the possibility that if we were pregnant there could be harm to the foetus.

For the last point there are some compelling reasons for caution. A 2020 report, *First Do No Harm*, by the UK's Baroness Cumberlege and her team looked at the impact of two medications and a medical device on women and their offspring.[27] The first was a type of hormone pregnancy test (HPT) given to women from the 1950s to the 1970s. It was seen as a quick and effective alternative to a long wait for the results of urine tests that, in those days, were sent off to a lab and injected in to mice, rabbits and frogs. If the first two ovulated or the frog spawned the result was positive, the woman was pregnant.

Unfortunately, none of the 'injectees' lived to tell the tale as the results were obtained on autopsy, leading to the euphemism 'the rabbit died' as a way to tell people they were pregnant. The HPTs involved women taking tablets that contained synthetic hormones (norethisterone and ethinyl estradiol) to induce a period-like bleed. If no bleeding occurred, the test was positive. But by the late 70s the drug was increasingly associated with birth defects and miscarriages and it was withdrawn.

The second was sodium valproate, a drug that works well for epilepsy but was associated with physical malformations, autism and developmental delay in some children if taken by their mothers during pregnancy.

The third was pelvic mesh implants that were used to help manage prolapses and stress urinary incontinence but ended up causing many women to endure 'crippling, life-changing, complications'. While this didn't cause birth defects the fact that these women endured unbearable pain that was often dismissed or passed off as 'part of menopause' is unforgivable and shows just how ingrained misogyny is in the health system.

All of these travesties, the report found, had a devastating effect on the women, children and families involved who had to fight for years to get recognition and compensation.

But they weren't isolated cases. Another scandal dating back to the 1950s and early 1960s involved the drug thalidomide. These days it's used to treat multiple myeloma and skin lesions in leprosy, but at that time it was given to help relieve morning sickness. It was prescribed to pregnant women in 49 different countries including the UK, Canada, Australia and New Zealand. It wasn't approved by the FDA in the US but it was given to 600 pregnant women in a trial.[28]

Back then they didn't know that drugs could cross the placental barrier to the baby, but it did, and if it was taken between days 20 and 37 of a pregnancy, a critical window for certain aspects of foetal development, it could cause limb deformities, sight and hearing loss as well as damage to internal organs. It was withdrawn in 1961, lawsuits followed and eventually compensation was paid. The first tranche was in 1968 amounting to £28 million in the UK and a further £20 million was paid by the government in 2009 to help cover the victim's costs.[29] In 2014, some 50 years later, the company that owns the UK manufacturer who supplied the Australian and New Zealand markets agreed to pay compensation to those victims to the tune of AU$89 million.[30]

No one likes to make a pay out, obviously, and the result was a considerable loss of appetite to include any women, pregnant or otherwise, in any clinical trials. It culminated in the FDA issuing a policy in 1977 recommending that women of childbearing age – that is all women aged 18 to around 50 – be excluded entirely from both the first two phases of clinical drug trials.[31]

When HIV arrived on the scene in the early 1980s, calls started for women to be allowed back into drug trials and in 1987 the National Institutes of Health (NIH), the main government-funded body for research in the US, issued a Guide for Grants and Contracts encouraging researchers to include women again.

A few years later the US Government Accountability Office (GAO) took a look at the NIH's record on getting more women into studies and found this had not been a great success. It discovered the funds were mainly used to pay for what's known as 'extramural research', that is, to help pay for salaries or research expenses rather than studies on women themselves. As a result, the NIH set up the Office of Research on Women's Health (ORWH) and in 1991 the infamous Women's Health Initiative (WHI) was born – the largest, and sometimes controversial, ongoing study on women ever launched. But it still wasn't a requirement to include women in clinical trials. This didn't happen for another couple of years when Congress added a section called 'Women and Minorities as Subjects in Clinical Research' to the NIH Revitalisation Act of 1993.[32]

Why the focus on the US? Because the budget for medical research in the US is huge compared to other countries. In 2024 it was just under $47.7 billion.[33] In the UK its equivalent, the National Institute for Health and Care Research (NIHR), spent £1.249 billion (US$1.667) in 2022–23.[34] Just putting that into perspective – the US population is about 335 million, the UK's is 70 million or about five times smaller, roughly, which means the US government is spending about 28 times more on research than the UK per head. In terms of GDP the US is around eight times larger, according to 2023 World Bank data, yet it is spending a significantly higher proportion on research than the UK – about 3.49 times more.[35]

In both the US and the UK, women are still underrepresented in research. Even though we're around 51 per cent of the population we make up anywhere between 29 and 44 per cent of the participants, depending on which study you look at. This is the case even when the conditions being studied are ones in which women bear a greater burden of disease, such as oncology, neurology, immunology and nephrology. A 2021 study published in the *JAMA Network Open* looked at 20,020 clinical trials involving more than five million participants and found that clinical trials for treatments in these areas had the lowest female representation even though women were more likely to be affected.[36]

Another in *Contemporary Clinical Trials* looked at cardiovascular disease and psychiatry studies involving more than 302,000 participants and found that for cardiovascular disease women made up 41.2 per cent of the cohort even though 49 per cent of the female population are affected by it.[37] For psychiatry the gap was even bigger. Some 60 per cent of psychiatric patients are women but just 42 per cent of the trial participants were women. The authors wrote: 'For each therapeutic area analyzed, the participation of females in clinical trials fell short of the benchmark derived from national prevalence data . . . Given potential sex-based differences in treatment responses and toxicities, adequate inclusion of females in clinical trials remains critical.' And when it comes to diversity, White women dominate the pool, making up around 75 per cent of participants.[38]

But there seems to be yet another reason for excluding women from trials that's currently emerging – gender politics. Commenting in *Time* magazine on the slow progress in including women, Dr Marianne Legato, Emerita Professor of Clinical Medicine at Columbia University and founder and director of the Foundation for Gender Specific Medicine, said: 'Many investigators are reluctant to emphasize sex differences in their research because of the emotional turmoil surrounding the evolving complexity of what gender means and what sex means. It's one of the elephants in the room of why gender-based research or male–female differences are not being more courageously investigated.'[39]

In other words, they're having difficulty separating sex at birth with sexual identity and as such, some (around 4 per cent of trials) aren't reporting on the sex of their participants at all, which means they won't show any data on what the adverse effects on women were. And as we've seen from the adverse events and stent example previously, not all drugs and devices work equally well in men and women.

The recent changes in the US on diversity, equity and inclusion (DEI) are not great news on this front either. Under the Biden administration draft guidelines were being prepared by the FDA to encourage researchers and pharma companies to include more people of colour and women in trials. Now with the purge of pages that contain any reference to DEI from government websites, including the FDA and the NIH, it's unclear what will happen to those guidelines. A recent decision to cut the WHI, which fortunately had a last-minute reprieve, would have been a huge blow to women's health.

When it comes to female participation in studies in the UK, the NIHR says it is behind the US, Canada and the EU, all of whom have made greater headway since the 1990s. But it says it's started to address this and the lack of diversity in studies with a series of initiatives designed to see more women and people from different ethnic or minority groups included.[40]

The double whammy – gender plus race

When it comes to 'minority' groups, particularly people from the Black community, there are some significant obstacles to taking part in research studies that centre on trust. We know that women of African and Caribbean descent have worse vasomotor symptoms and, to add insult to injury, they have them for longer than their White counterparts. They may also go through menopause earlier than their White counterparts which may put them at higher risk of dementia and heart disease, so more research is a priority. But the history of mistreatment and abuse of Black people by the medical establishment, and in clinical trials, means trust must be rebuilt and that's going to take some doing.

You might think we're harking back to centuries-old abuse here, but no, between 1932 and 1972 – yes, 1972 – various US government health bodies including today's Centers for Disease Control (CDC) ran a study that involved injecting 600 Black American men with syphilis and systematically lying to them for decades about what they were being treated for.[41] They also took active steps to ensure they didn't get the appropriate treatment, penicillin, by providing local doctors in their area with a list of trial participants and asking them not to treat them. It was known as the Tuskegee study, and its aim was to 'observe the natural history of untreated syphilis'. It was only finally stopped when a whistleblower leaked information about the trial to the *New York Times* in 1972.[42]

But it doesn't end there. In the 1960s, inmates of a Philadelphia prison, many of whom were Black, were subjected to tests that exposed them to high levels of dioxin, a known carcinogen. Between 1907 and 1979 around 20,000 women, mostly Black or 'women of colour' were forcibly sterilised. In North Carolina sterilisations of Black women were used to 'weed out any feeble minded'. In the 1990s an unethical US trial paid parents to enrol their Black American boys into a study that hypothesised that aggressive behaviour has a genetic base. The boys were given a drug that was associated with instigating aggressive behaviour and denied water and their medications, including asthma medications, during an overnight stay without their parents being present.

Then there's a long history of grave robbing to steal bodies to dissect, as well as slave owners selling the bodies of deceased slaves to medical schools.[43] And on top of that, there are the surgeries inflicted upon enslaved women by the 'father of gynaecology', J. Marion Sims, who spent his time between 1845 and 1849 experimenting on Black women who had a vaginal fistula as a result of childbirth. A vaginal fistula is a hole that develops in the birth canal which can result in urine or faeces passing though the vagina. It is an infection risk and can be fatal. Sims wanted to find a way to repair it, so experimented on Black slaves. Three of the women have been honoured now as the 'mothers of gynaecology' with statues erected in Alabama in their honour. One woman, Anarcha, endured at least 30 surgeries with no pain relief. Modern anaesthesia was introduced in 1846 with mixed results, but no forms of pain relief were offered to these women.[44]

These kinds of things stay with people, and trust is hard to restore once it's lost. It may go part way to explain why Black people only made up 5 per cent of the participants in the COVID vaccine trials even though they represent 14 per cent of the UK population and were almost twice as likely to die as their White counterparts if they contracted the virus.[45] This wasn't helped by false rumours, of course, claiming that Africans were used as guinea pigs for the vaccine trial and that people had died[46] or that the vaccine could cause sterility.[47]

Dr Itunuoluwa Johnson-Sogbetun, a GP with a special interest in menopause care and member of the Royal College of General Practitioners Northwest London Faculty Board, where she leads its equality, diversity and inclusion strategy, sees the impact of menopause on Black women's health all the time. She often meets women struggling with debilitating symptoms who are hesitant to consider MHT. 'This hesitation is not simply about personal preference; it is shaped by deep-rooted concerns including fears about breast cancer scare stories, feelings that these treatments are not "natural", distrust in the medical establishment, and the reality that Black women have been underrepresented in clinical trials. As a result, many women lack confidence that these treatments are safe or appropriate for them.'

Yet, she says, 'Black women are more likely to go through menopause around two years earlier than their White counterparts, are at greater risk of experiencing premature menopause, and often endure symptoms for up to four years longer. Without support, this prolonged and sometimes more severe menopausal experience can increase the risk of long-term health issues, including heart disease, osteoporosis and dementia. This is especially concerning as Black women are already at higher risk of developing cardiovascular risk factors such as hypertension, obesity and diabetes. These risks intersect with menopause to further increase the likelihood of poor health outcomes later in life. For symptomatic women, and particularly those experiencing early or premature menopause, MHT can play a crucial role in protecting heart and bone health, as well as improving quality of life.

'I understand the fears women have – especially when so much of the information about HRT feels confusing,' says Dr Johnson-Sogbetun. 'But for women who are struggling, and especially for Black women who face an earlier and often more difficult menopause, the evidence shows that the benefits of HRT – particularly for heart and bone health – often outweigh the risks. It can be life-changing for those experiencing severe symptoms.'

But she says the lack of trust is real and compounded by current day medical misogyny. 'Black women's concerns are often grounded in real experiences of being dismissed by healthcare professionals, coupled with cultural anxieties around menopause being seen as a loss of status, desirability, or value. Faith considerations can also come into play, with some women questioning whether HRT aligns with their Christian, Muslim, or traditional beliefs.'

She says, 'Women need to feel heard and respected. Conversations about menopause must recognise the diversity of Black women's experiences – what feels safe, what aligns with our values, and what supports our health span and quality of life.'

When a woman's health suffers so does their ability to stay in work, care for others and contribute fully to society. Investing in culturally competent menopause care and closing the research gaps that have left women behind is not just a matter of equity – it's an economic imperative. Supporting women's health means supporting their participation in work and community life, with benefits that ripple far beyond the individual.

But for progress to be made we need more research – a lot more. The leading causes of death and the conditions that reduce women's health span and quality of life – cardiovascular disease, dementia, bladder issues and incontinence, and osteoporosis – are all affected by menopause. Yet the role of menopause in these health outcomes remains under-researched and poorly understood. Dr Johnson-Sogbetun is clear: 'We cannot close the gaps in women's health until we close the gaps in the evidence. We need research that reflects the realities of all women – including Black women – so we can support longer, healthier lives.'

But it's not just the killer conditions that need more research. Investing in research on migraine/headaches, PMS, depressive disorder, causes of fatigue and chronic musculoskeletal pain as well as period pain, endometriosis and adenomyosis could massively reduce days off and boost the economy.

In the US, the Biden administration made some significant moves to improve the research into women's health and menopause. Spurred on by the collective efforts of campaigners like Maria Schriver, a Kennedy family member, former Californian 'first lady' and journalist; a group of 17 senators from both the Republican and Democratic parties; leading medical researchers; celebrities like Halle Berry, and former first lady Jill Biden, former president Biden issued an Executive Order calling on Congress to invest $12 billion in new funding for women's health research across the life span, including midlife and perimenopause and menopause.

The NIH itself is lifting its game too. It has launched an NIH-wide effort to close gaps in women's health, allocating $200 million of its 2025 budget to drive interdisciplinary, multi-faceted research projects on the impact of perimenopause and menopause on heart health, brain health and bone health.

Whether these initiatives survive the Trump administration, which has pledged to drive out the 'woke' policies from an organisation that he claims are 'pushing junk gender science',[48] remains to be seen, but Jennifer Weiss-Wolf is optimistic.

'It might be like a weird unicorn. I think it's going to stand out even more in the next two years, because abortion is going to be so polarising and so toxic. I think that this issue might win more attention from Republicans, who maybe will feel like they need to do some good deed on women's health, given that they're eviscerating it in other ways.'

The UK hasn't made quite the same commitment moneywise. The amount spent on women's health research in general, the NHS Confederation says, is about 2 per cent and that's remained static for a decade. It's called for ringfenced funding for the *Women's Health Strategy*, additional funding for the NIHR for women's health research to promote understanding of, and treatment options for, conditions that solely affect women, including menopause. It also recommended that the government continue to fund women's health hubs across England to help deliver treatments and services in a primary care setting. These hubs were a key plank of the ten-year *Women's Health Strategy* but were only funded for two years. That's not really a lot of time to show how well they've performed. The money was available to all 42 regions in England and by the end of 2024, 36 of them had set up a hub providing various women's health services. Not all, however, provide menopause services. The NHS Confederation estimated the return on investment for every £1 spent on these would be £5, but without a commitment to long-term funding that will be difficult to realise, the authors wrote.[49]

The Confederation has called for a commitment to an annual 1 per cent increase in overall public research funding that is dedicated to 'reproductive health and childbirth'. And it wants to know how much of that is allocated to maternity versus gynaecology services, as well as those conditions we mentioned before that affect women disproportionately.

It's not all bad news though. There has been some positive movement on menopause research in the UK with the 2022 *Women's Health Strategy* through the NIHR commissioning research into menopause, including a £2.2 million randomised control trial looking at the effectiveness of different hormone treatments for women with Premature Ovarian Insufficiency.[50] And the NIHR has also announced £2.6 million to fund a study into reported beneficial effects of testosterone beyond low libido.

Ultimately, we have a long way to get parity, but any dollar or pound spent today will undoubtedly save money and improve lives tomorrow, as well as boosting the economy considerably.

6

Show me the money – Policy, politics and menopause products

'You're worth it!' Oh yes you are – in fact, you're worth around $15 trillion, and that's just counting American women over 50. According to *Forbes* magazine, America's 40 million or so women in their 50s 'represent over $15 trillion in purchasing power and are the healthiest, wealthiest, and most active generation in history. This group of super consumers, who will experience the largest population growth over the next 10 years, represent off-the-charts spending power, yet most of these women feel completely ignored by marketers.'[1]

Well, not anymore. You and your peri-and-menoposse pals around the world are now firmly in the sights of the menopause marketers and you are literally their dream come true. You've gained weight, you're anxious, your moods are insane, your skin and hair are shot, your bladder betrays you with every step you take and your vagina is so dry it makes the Sahara look like a luxury oasis retreat (but, thankfully, your libido is as dead as a dodo anyway, so it doesn't really matter!)

But fear not, there's something for each of these ailments, and let's face it there's nothing that stops you in your morning social media scroll faster than an orgasming middle-aged woman with a tube of rose-scented lube in her hand doing a *When Harry Met Sally* impersonation in a diner. (Please don't buy scented lube. You *really* don't want what she's having.) In any case, if you hadn't noticed, the market for menopause products is big. In 2024 the global market was valued at $17.66 billion and it's expected to grow to $27.63 billion by 2033,[2] and you walking wodges of cash are manna from heaven because there's nothing a marketer loves more than a vulnerable woman who's ready to be empowered with one click of a 'buy now' button.

And you're already haemorrhaging cash. In fact, at $103/month, US-based menopausal women spend the most of all groups on products, according to a 2024 McKinsey report, on wellness trends.[3] Pregnancy-related products come in second at $96/month.

Why are you parting with your hard-earned cash? You're 'Taking back control,' 'balancing hormones', 'boosting energy', 'clearing brain fog', 'flattening your meno belly' so you can 'make your husband go WOAH!'[4] – that's not a joke, by the way, it's from a real ad.

None of this is new to Professor Samantha Thomas; she's seen it all before. She has a truly interesting job looking at the impact corporations have on the health, wellbeing or health inequity within populations. Based at the Faculty of Health, Institute for Health Transformation at Deakin University in Australia, she's studied how the alcohol, tobacco and gambling industries work and is now casting an eye over the sales tactics being used in the menopause market and says they are remarkably familiar. 'We know that some population groups are more vulnerable to the harms associated with the tactics or playbooks of these industries. Children and young people would be one, and women are the other group.'

Initially women fly underneath the radar with these industries until they need to expand their customer base and that's when they 'develop products and use strategies to bring women in. So, if we think about the alcohol industry's "pink washing" of products, or the tobacco industry's use of empowerment messages. And we're seeing the gambling industry using things around glamour and feminism. All of those strategies are particularly used to engage a female market.'

It's something the diet industry has excelled at, Thomas says, playing 'on women's fears and body image to become a huge billion-dollar business. And I think what we're seeing at the moment is a similar sort of thing happening with menopause. You have something that has been framed as taboo or stigmatised, or something that we don't really talk about. And then we have a whole lot of people jumping on to that and using these "empowerment models".'

Veteran Australian journalist turned academic and author of four books looking at the business of medicine over the past few decades, Ray Moynihan says this is a favourite tactic employed by the pharmaceutical industry too across a range of conditions. 'There is growing evidence that medical companies are co-opting the language of feminism and emancipation and empowerment . . . Pharma marketing deliberately tries to blur the lines between normal and sick because there is a lot of money to be made convincing healthy people they are sick', or in this case, that the ever-expanding list of menopause symptoms need treating.

An example Thomas cites for menopause is the use of the 'gaslighting narrative'. Yes, it's true that women are gaslit (see Chapter 4) but in this case she says it has created an opportunity for marketers across the board to capitalise on by 'stepping in to give women a solution'.

And the polarised views aren't helping. 'We've got these two competing framings of menopause going on: women are no longer useful, they're irrational, unstable and grumpy all the time, or, it's a natural, normal part of the ageing process. And some of this framing is coming from really powerful groups and institutions. Some are coming from the medical profession and some are from commercial entities who are seeking to profit from menopause. And we've got some framing coming from the media and the government, and that creates a really confusing messaging environment for women. They're left wondering; who do I believe?'

Enter another form of influencer, not the celebrity or medical influencer, but 'real women', and they have a unique advantage. 'Quite often you trust recognised celebrities. You would see them as being similar to you, very trustworthy. But celebrities are slightly different from you, or distant from you, whereas the influencers bring you into their community. So, for women who might be feeling a bit isolated or alone or misunderstood, suddenly you feel part of something. You feel connected to something.' But the problem is 'there are many different types of influencers and it's very difficult for women to navigate what's accurate information that's supported by robust evidence, and what's not'.

The other question is – are they being paid to deliver a certain message? Professor Thomas says it's a very muddy space. When it comes to influencers in the UK, the Advertising Standards Association (ASA) states that influencers have to make clear if they are being paid in any way to promote a product, and that includes getting free goods. Ideally the ASA wants them to display the word 'AD' clearly on any post at the start, but it's virtually impossible to police and very few do declare it. How do I know? Because I've watched more of them than I care to remember. They talk about a problem, how 'X' could fix it or be worth trying, or has done wonders for them and often give a discount code or directions to an affiliate website – but nowhere on the post do they say it was a paid promotion, sponsored post let alone 'ad'. Sometimes you may see '#gifted' – but what does that tell you?

Celebrity endorsements of a product are usually pretty obvious and many are very good at saying it's a 'sponsored post', but what about when they're just talking about their own experiences and how awful menopause had been and how much certain treatments may have helped them? Thomas says this catastrophising is another tactic that's used to drive sales and studies show it works.[5] So when a celebrity says she was wrecked by anxiety or insomnia and then says what helped her, it's impossible to know if she's been paid to say it or not. She would like to see robust regulations governing the declaration of payments made to celebrities and influencers in general, to ensure there is transparency.

The next question is – are all these meno-magnets, face creams, shampoos, supplements and devices that promise to relieve your symptoms and transform your life actually worth paying for?

Do you need them and do they work?

We know people are spending huge amounts every month on all types of menopause supplements. The BBC *Panorama* programme that looked at the industry spoke to UK women who were outspending the Americans, forking out around £150 a month on products that claim to help with symptoms. A recent Clearpay survey came up with about the same figure annually (£1,800) being spent mostly on vitamins, minerals, shampoos and skincare products.[6] I've spoken to doctors who say women turn up in their clinics with shopping bags full of pills and potions – so many that they're surprised that they can't hear the women themselves rattling as they come through the door. I remember one woman telling me she'd bought a magnet that sticks in your underwear to relieve her symptoms. Unfortunately, the only benefit it provided was a hands-free shopping experience at the supermarket because the trolley snapped happily onto her waist.

So, do you really need these products? Let's look at vitamins first. Most doctors and dieticians say that unless you have a deficiency you should be able to get pretty much all you need from your diet.

One exception is vitamin D. You can get a bit from your diet, but you really need a bit of daily sun exposure to make this, so if you live in a cold climate, don't get outside much or are well covered when you do, you may need a supplement. Public Health England says we should take a vitamin D supplement from October to April. It recommends 400IU a day but many doctors say 800IU a day is a better mark to aim for. If you have darker skin you may need to take more than your fair-skinned friends, but speak to your doctor to see what's right for you.

Vitamin D is essential for bone health, muscles, brain function and immune systems. But an important thing to remember is that vitamin D is fat soluble – that means it's stored in your fat and not peed out like an excess of vitamin C would be. So, unless you've been told by your doctor you need more, don't think 'if a little bit is good, more must be better', because too much of it can be bad for your bones, kidneys and heart. You can always get a base level from a blood test, so ask your doctor. If you are deficient you will need to take enough to correct that, and they can advise on how much and for how long.

Two extremely down-to-earth dieticians who work with a lot of menopausal women are Elizabeth Ward and Hillary Wright in the US. They're the authors of the *Menopause Diet Plan* and they spend a lot of time debunking weight loss, diet and supplement myths. When it comes to other supplements they say 'food first'. Despite what we're told by advertisers most people are not deficient in vitamins and minerals but 'it depends on their diet and where they are in the menopause transition,' Ward says. For example, 'if a woman is perimenopausal and has heavy periods, she may also need some extra iron, which should be determined with her doctor,' she adds. 'With any supplement, it's important to think of them as a way to bridge gaps between what's in your diet and the recommended intakes,' or RDIs. You can get a blood test from your doctor to assess your iron levels. Ferritin is the thing to look out for and UK guidelines suggest it should be above 30 mcg/litre, below that and you are considered deficient.[7] Most of the doctors I've spoken to over the years say they'd like to see it above 60 mcg/litre. You need it to be higher if you're pregnant. Again, it's another one that you don't want to go overboard on as too much can damage the kidneys. Some labs say the maximum should be around 200 mcg/litre.

Here is Ward's take on some of the commonly recommended supplements for menopausal women:

- Calcium – Some women may need extra, for example 'if I get only 600 milligrams of calcium every day in food, then I should take 600 milligrams to satisfy the suggested intake of 1,200 milligrams a day. Taking more isn't going to prevent me from getting osteoporosis and it may mess up the balance of nutrients in the body.' There is no proof that taking more can help your heart or bone health, she says, and it may have some downsides.[8] The NHS advises that taking too much, more than 1,500mg/day in a supplement, may cause stomach upsets and diarrhoea.[9] Hypercalcaemia may occur with excessive doses or if you have a hyperparathyroid condition and this can affect heart and kidney function and in extreme cases can be life-threatening.[10] There are some apps that can help you track the amount of calcium you are getting.
- Multivitamins – Research suggests 'that taking a garden-variety multivitamin every day slows brain aging'[11] (but other research shows they add very little to longevity[12]).
- Magnesium (mg) for sleep – 'Some people swear by magnesium glycinate for sleep, but there's no research that shows it works.'
- Valerian – 'is another supplement that may be effective for sleep, and so is melatonin.' (Melatonin is only available on prescription in the UK, and for short-term use. It is not suitable for people with autoimmune conditions, or liver or kidney problems.)
- Omega-3 – 'Women who don't eat fatty fish, such as salmon, at least twice weekly will need omega-3 supplements.' (Other sources of omega-3s are sardines, mackerel, anchovies and some seeds and nuts like flax seeds, chia seeds and walnuts.)

It is worth remembering that supplements are not approved by regulatory bodies or tested for effectiveness, but unless they make outrageous claims little notice is taken of them. There are very few quality controls and when studies have been done to look at whether they contain what they say they do, discrepancies have been found. One study of products claiming to boost memory in the US found that two of the three tested did not contain the amount of the active ingredient they stated, and in one it couldn't be detected at all. Some contained contaminants like arsenic or chromium.[13] It's been estimated that around 23,000 admissions to hospital in the US are related to supplements[14] and one in 55 admissions is related to an adverse reaction between a prescribed medication and a supplement, according to Israeli research.[15] So, make sure your doctor knows what you're taking.

How do you know what to look for then?

Ward says: 'We recommend sticking with the big, well-established companies because they have a longstanding presence in the market and generally don't add much else besides vitamins and minerals to their supplements. The "recipe" for combining vitamins and minerals often requires some stabilisers and fillers so that nutrients don't interact with each other and to keep them from disintegrating. Avoid supplements with extra herbs and other botanicals, though. They add cost with no guarantee of effectiveness. In the US, supplements are not regulated like drugs so it's difficult to know what you're getting in an herbal supplement, whether it's contaminated with a heavy metal, or if it will be effective, but I trust the big companies because they have a lot more to lose than smaller, fly-by-night internet companies.

'My extra comment is stay away from so-called "experts" who have designed their own supplements. There is no need for designer supplements – it's not as if these people have discovered some secret knowledge about vitamins and minerals. Designer supplements are usually far more expensive and no more effective than what you buy at the pharmacy.'

Some products say they are manufactured to Good Manufacturing Practices standards (GMP) or have a label saying 'THR' which stands for 'Traditional Herbal Remedy'. A THR seal shows the ingredients have been used for 30 years or more, it is not a guarantee of the quality of the product itself. The FDA says GMP seals 'do not guarantee that a product is safe or effective' – only that the products should contain what they say they do.[16]

The take-home message – food first

But if you buy a supplement, for example, to help you sleep or to reduce your anxiety and it does no harm and you can afford it, then it's your money, your choice, go crazy! Just make sure your doctor knows what you're taking as some 'natural' supplements can interact with other medicines. And if you're taking multiple things – this is really important – have a look at the amounts of each ingredient they contain as you don't want to be doubling up on things and end up taking too much of something by accident. If they don't show the amount of the ingredients they contain – don't take them. Manufacturers in the UK are required to list the amount of the ingredients in their products, any potential allergens, and their contact details, among other things.[17] You can look up Recommended Daily Intake (RDI) charts to see how much of a vitamin or mineral you should have and then compare it to the amount in the products you are taking. And remember you may already have enough from your diet.

What about products that claim to help with vasomotor symptoms?

When it comes to hot flushes and night sweats specifically, there are a lot of products that claim to relieve them, but a huge meta-analysis done by the Menopause Society in the US of non-hormonal treatments found none of those they looked at had enough data behind them to back the claims.[18] I know this may be disappointing for some, but they found no good evidence for all of the following:

- Cooling techniques like facial sprays, cool pillows, fans, cold packs for the neck
- Avoiding triggers like spicy food, alcohol or caffeine
- Yoga (sorry! Stress maybe; hot flushes, no)
- Changing your diet
- Mindfulness
- Relaxation or breathing techniques
- Soy or soy metabolites (isoflavones that bind to oestrogen receptors)
- Pollen extracts
- Ammonium succinate

- Lactobacillus acidophilus
- Siberian rhubarb
- Black cohosh
- Wild yam – yes, it's used to synthesise the oestrogen in the prescription medications but there's no evidence that eating it or putting it in a cream will make any difference to vasomotor symptoms
- Dong quai
- Evening primrose
- Maca
- Ginseng
- Chasteberry (*agnus castus*)
- Milk thistle
- Omega-3
- Vitamin E
- Cannabinoids (CBD)

What did work for vasomotor symptoms when it came to non-hormonal and non-medical treatments was weight loss, cognitive behavioural therapy (CBT) and hypnosis. These last two are not implying that the symptoms are 'all in your head' but giving you different strategies to deal with them.

Many people may disagree with the list above and swear by the supplements they take, and if it does no harm and you're happy – again, it's your money, your choice. Again, just make sure your doctor knows what you're taking.

None of this commercialisation would be such an issue, Jennifer Weiss-Wolf says, 'if people could go to their doctors and get answers and get prescriptions, if prescriptions were easier to get or more affordable. All of those things would stymie the commercial market, because people would really be more empowered and less confused and wouldn't have to rely on these, but then, because this is the world we live in, people are being tricked. And it makes me mad when friends say, "Oh, I bought this supplement, and I bought this cream and I bought this whatever," when you just really needed a little tube of vaginal oestrogen for vaginal dryness, but they don't know that. And then when the celebrities make a lot of money off it, it irritates me.'

And she's especially irritated when there are false claims involved. 'In the case of the United States, there's an agency called the Federal

Trade Commission that could be a lot more robust in terms of cracking down on false claims, or could publish perhaps a glossary so people could wade through all the fake terms that are used or posted, what kinds of claims to steer clear of so consumers can be more discerning. Those are the things that we could do to ameliorate the commercial market a little bit.'

Such claims might include terms like 'oestrogen dominant', 'hormone balancing', 'helps burn meno belly fat', 'natural and safer than hormones', or things like 'backed by science', or 'clinically proven' when no independent, quality trials are provided other than those done by the manufacturer themselves.

For Diane Danzebrink many of these products that aren't backed by good science and are proof positive that the 'greedy genie' is out of the bottle and playing havoc in the market. 'We have to accept that menopause is now very much an industry . . . When you are seeing things like menopause shampoo, menopause chocolate, and countless menopause supplements coming to the market it's clear that ultimately this is about exploitation and I hate it. But, money makes the world go round and where there is money to be made, I honestly don't see that there will be any reduction in the marketing or advertising of these products, or any serious clipping of the wings of those who sell them. My advice to everyone is buyer beware, do your due diligence, it could save you a lot of money.'

Vagina cream on your face? It's a thing

You may remember earlier on we discussed the 1960s and the delightful statements from Robert Wilson's book *Feminine Forever* that menopausal women were 'castrates' whose breasts and genitals shrivel while they become 'dull and unattractive' unless they're on MHT. Then came Lauren Hutton in the late 1990s/early 2000s in a paid ad saying she could spot women on hormones because they didn't look 'shrunk or dried up'. Well, here we are a quarter of a century later and we're being told to put our vaginal cream on our face – or pay a hefty sum for a cream that's actually made for our faces with oestrogen in it. For those who are asking 'what, what vaginal cream?' there are various products prescribed to treat the Genitourinary Syndrome of

Menopause (GSM) and one is a cream that usually contains a form of oestrogen called estriol (see Chapter 9). So, how far have we come? Not very, it seems. Hormone therapy is still being touted as the 'elixir of youth'. Which is fine, if that's what you want, but remember there are marketing forces at play here that are subtly (well, perhaps not so subtly) reinforcing the youth-oriented culture while simultaneously and possibly unwittingly promoting ageism – that is, you're only of value if you still look young.

Studies looking at the 'pinkification' of the menopause marketplace – that is, products directed to menopausal women – show there are four standard tropes that are used to get us to press that 'buy' button.[19]

They are:

1 *The return* – a promise, often with empowering language like 'youth restored, confidence ignited', 'glow young, feel strong' or the familiar 'you're worth it' – that tell you can 'reclaim' your lost youth.
2 *Girly sexuality* – unless you're young, skinny and flawless, you're worthless, but we can help you get that back (like 'flatten that belly and make your husband go "woah"' that I mentioned before).
3 *Calming and quietening* – you're menopausal, you're hysterical and can't cope – but we can fix that.
4 *Brain boosting* – that brain fog is doing your head in, but we have the solution that will keep you on your game and boost your productivity. You'll be employee of the month in no time!

Dr Hannah Swift, Reader in Social and Organisational Psychology at the University of Kent, who looks at ageism in society and workplaces, says 'we live in a world that values youth over old age and it's deeply entrenched in media. If you look at any fashion magazine, everything's orientated towards youth' and this is a tough attitude to overcome with deep cultural and evolutionary roots. In work she's done looking at the fashion industry, Swift says there's been a bit of movement with older women appearing more often and the #NoMoreWrinklyHands campaign was quite useful in pushing things along. It questioned why, as its name suggests, older people were often represented by wrinkly hands and called for more diversity when it comes to the images chosen to depict people from midlife onwards. But the online world is yet to catch up, she says. 'There's been a slight change there with a few older influencers, but even they get quite a lot of backlash or negative trolling.'

There sure is! Personal trainer Kate Oakley, founder of Your Future Fit, has borne the brunt of it with negative comments like 'stop flashing your old lady body on social media', 'aged 54, isn't it time you ditched the bikinis', 'you look 70' and 'stop lifting weights and exercise appropriately for your age' – all of which she shrugged off with a polite 'No!' But once again, it shows how others' opinions can pressure us to conform to the stereotype of what ageing should look like – disappearing quietly into the furniture.

This type of gendered ageism is more than just nasty, it can be damaging, Swift says. 'Ageism or any kind of prejudice is called a psychological stressor. It creates a stress response in people and it damages confidence and self-esteem.'

But, if we slap on that oestrogen cream all our wrinkles will disappear within weeks – restoration complete! Much of this has come from the US where they can advertise prescription products directly to consumers, and not surprisingly those who are selling the creams are huge enthusiasts. But do they work? The logic is, if it works for the vagina it should work for the face. There are some studies, mostly small and short term, that show that putting a cream that contains oestrogen on your face could improve collagen and elastin production and the result would be firmer and thicker-looking skin. And when I say small studies, I'm talking 60 people or fewer. Other studies have shown it has no effect on sun-damaged skin and let's face it (no pun intended) that's pretty much everyone who's been outside – in fact it found it caused an increase in an enzyme that increases the breakdown of collagen.[20] (To be fair it was using estrone, a different type of oestrogen that is not the type being used in the other creams.)

Is it safe? We're told that it's safe for our vagina, so surely it must be OK to take an extra bit of that cream you've been prescribed for your vagina and slap it on your face? Some of the studies show there is little systemic absorption when used in a specific area as in a square on the buttock, which was one area studied, and one industry-funded study but conducted by an independent lab shows there was a non-significant increase in absorption of their product when used on the face for 12 weeks.[21] The protocol here was 'apply 3 pumps (approximately 1 ml of product) to face (forehead, cheeks, under/ around eyes) and neck at bedtime after cleansing'.

But some experts question whether you're really going to limit it to your face and neck when your décolletage and hands have craters in them that are deeper than the Grand Canyon?

Australian GP and author of *The M Word*, Dr Ginni Mansberg isn't convinced you will. She has a skincare line which does not sell oestrogen-based products, so you may argue she's biased against it, but she's spent years scouring journals looking at evidence-backed ingredients that are safe and effective. She concedes these studies, that usually look at estradiol, show that it can improve hydration and boost collagen and elastin but questions why some of the face products are using estriol – a weaker form of oestrogen that's made by the placenta. It is the type usually used in topical creams for vaginal dryness. And it works, but it's worth remembering that the vagina has a mucosal lining which is not the same as the keratinised, thicker skin on your face.

'My concerns are the following. We know that oestrogen is absorbed across the skin, and it is the preferred way that we deliver oestrogen to menopausal women. So, once we know that 1) it's absorbed by the skin, and that 2) it's in a form that comes out of the placenta, my concern is how much do you need to put on your skin, not the vagina, but the skin, because most of the studies of this around safety have been done on vaginal delivery of estriol cream. The risks are that we increase your risk of endometrial thickening and the potential for vaginal bleeding and the potential for what we call endometrial hyperplasia, so an overgrowth of the endometrium. So, at what point do we need to give you progesterone?'

Thirdly, she says, 'the amount we use in the vagina is half a milli-litre but that isn't going to be enough to cover your entire face, neck, décolletage or the backs of your hands' and, unlike vaginal cream which most women use twice a week, you'd be using it on your face every day. 'We don't have good safety data for using large amounts of estriol. Does it behave in the same way when it's absorbed transder-mally? We don't really know, because we don't have good long-term follow-up studies. It might be totally fine, and studies would suggest that it will be rejuvenating to the skin of the face, so let's not say it's not going to work. We think it probably will, but we'd need larger studies to confirm safety rather than efficacy.'

And, if you're using it on both ends, your face and genitalia, Mansberg says there are no studies on that as yet. Proponents say it's a tiny amount in these creams so in theory shouldn't pose a problem. But, we don't know.

So, that's a 'no' from her, for the time being at least. If you really want to help the skin on your face a daily sunscreen is a must, and vitamins A (retinol/retinal/tretinoin) and C (L-ascorbic acid) and niacinamide (B3) have good evidence behind them. And looking after your skin is important as we age, and not just on our faces, our bodies matter too (see Chapter 10).

But what about shampoos or face creams which claim they're specifically made for menopausal women? Mansberg is pretty clear on her view saying it's 'frank exploitation of women. No, you don't need a menopause-specific skincare product. No, your face would not fall off if you were a man and used it, nor would your face fall off if you were a 20-year-old. We don't have the evidence for menopause-specific supplements or menopause-specific skincare.'

But her real ire falls on the purveyors of compounded bio-identical hormone products known as cBHT in US or bHRT in the UK. These are products that are often touted as being 'safer' than the MHT your doctor will give you. They often require expensive urine, saliva or blood tests that need to be repeated regularly, and boast that they're tailor-made for your specific needs. They are not endorsed by any menopause society across the globe because they haven't been tested for safety or efficacy. Because they are compounded by private pharmacies they aren't regulated so you don't really know if you're getting what you paid for. The FDA has issued a warning about them saying 'there is limited federal and state-level oversight of the quality and use of cBHT preparations. Given the lack of high-quality clinical evidence and minimal oversight of cBHT, [the National Academies of Science, Engineering, and Medicine] NASEM concluded that their widespread use poses a public health concern.'[22] These are mostly offered in private clinics and Mansberg is concerned that the menopause societies aren't doing enough to stop their spread, concentrating their energies instead on the 'medical influencers' while letting another horse bolt before their noses.

An untasty toastie

It's not just claims made about supplements that need stronger regulations. There is a burgeoning industry for home testing kits and home use devices. The home testing kits offer the ability to tell you where you are on your 'menopause journey' by measuring your Follicle Stimulating Hormone (FSH – the one that makes the ovaries produce an egg) in either your blood or urine. Nice idea but there's no validation for the urine test and it's unlikely that your doctor will accept the results from either the home-bought urine or blood test because it hasn't come from a lab that they accept results from. They don't know if it's kosher or not. Plus, if you're over 45, you're diagnosed on symptoms, not blood test results, so don't waste your money. Both the British Menopause Society (BMS) and the Royal College of Obstetricians and Gynaecologist (RCOG) recommend speaking to your doctor instead – which will cost you nothing in the UK at least.

These aren't the only things being offered for home use. You may have noticed that vaginal rejuvenation using laser or radiofrequency devices is being offered by some clinics. They claim it can improve bladder function, vaginal dryness and give your sex life a boost as well. The jury is still out on the effectiveness of these energy-based devices like CO_2 fractional laser or radiofrequency, with some independent studies showing laser treatments are no better than a sham (or a fake treatment),[23] but others showing they may be a useful part of the armamentarium for relieving vaginal dryness, and others saying more evidence is needed.[24,25,26]

The Australian Therapeutic Goods Administration (TGA) isn't buying any of it though and has 'cancelled' all vaginal rejuvenation products from its list of registered therapeutic goods after a review which said 'there was insufficient clinical evidence to support the therapeutic use and long-term safety of these devices'.[27] That's a major blow to the industry down under, and means those very expensive machines can no longer be imported or exported from the country.

Clinic treatments are one thing, but now you can bypass those and buy home use devices online. At the click of a button you can have it discreetly delivered – and then 'plug and play'.

Some of these devices heat the tissue in the vagina to around 42–65 degrees Celsius (65 degrees – that's heading towards egg-cooking hot!), and some have a vibrating mode as well, as a 'bonus extra'.[28] So, here's the thing – or things:

- They may say they are FDA approved – but they are not. The FDA has not (as of writing) approved laser or radiofrequency for vaginal rejuvenation. It has, in fact, issued a warning against using these devices except for approved purposes which are for the removal of genital warts or pre-cancerous lesions. Why? Because the safety and efficacy hasn't been established. This is what it wrote in 2018 when these devices came on the market for clinic use – before you could buy them for home use:

  > In reviewing adverse event reports and published literature, we have found numerous cases of vaginal burns, scarring, pain during sexual intercourse, and recurring or chronic pain. We haven't reviewed or approved these devices for use in such procedures. Thus, the full extent of the risks is unknown. But these reports indicate these procedures can cause serious harm. Today, we're warning women and their healthcare providers that the FDA has serious concerns about the use of these devices to treat gynecological [sic] conditions beyond those for which the devices have been approved or cleared.[29]

  So, if the clinic versions haven't been given the FDA the all-clear it would be highly unlikely that the home use ones have.
- Heating your vaginal tissue while you're enjoying that bonus vibrator means you're probably not going to use it as directed, so you're at risk of slowly toasting your vaginal mucosa.
- If you have not had an assessment to check what is causing your issues in the first place you could be missing out on a treatment that you actually need, and you may even make the condition you have worse.
- Independent studies to show these home use devices are safe or effective are few and far between (think hen's teeth) and are usually done by or paid for by the manufacturer.

- A 'CE mark' or 'UKCA mark' shows that the device complies with EU or UK health and safety requirements – so it won't electrocute you when you turn it on. It is not an MHRA endorsement of safety and efficacy as a treatment. The MHRA says: 'A UKCA mark is a logo that is placed on medical devices to show they conform to the requirements in the UK MDR 2002. It shows that the device is fit for its intended purpose stated and meets legislation relating to safety.'[30]

If you want to search to see if a product has a medical device registration in the UK there is a MHRA Public Access Registration Database – and it clearly states, 'Registration of medical devices with the MHRA (the UK Competent Authority) does not represent any form of accreditation, certification, approval or endorsement by the MHRA.'[31]

A quick trip to online shops shows some of these devices make unbelievable claims like 'treating cervical erosion, cervicitis, mild non-specific vaginitis and vaginal contraction. Restore your normal intimate balance levels at the same time.' The last sentence doesn't even make sense, and if you have some of these conditions you need medical attention, a proper diagnosis and a prescribed treatment. Others claim to cure 'abnormal menstrual bleeding', 'vaginal foreign bodies' (I guess that depends on what exactly the foreign body is), and 'cervical erosion'.[32] This latter one usually resolves on its own but if it doesn't it needs treatment by a medical professional. This falls firmly into the 'do not try this at home' category.

FiFi's Fabulous Fannies

Now, at risk of sounding like a travelling salesman about to throw in a set of steak knives to close the deal, let me just say – it doesn't end there.

In researching for moderating a panel discussion on the regulations needed in this market, I decided I would contact the manufacturers of some of the devices being offered to clinics. I found some in China who were advertising laser devices for sale at around £8,000 – that's about £50,000 cheaper than the devices you'd usually find in a reputable clinic. I told them I was a hairdresser, and I was interested in putting one into my salon. They said no problem, and they could send one of their beauticians to train me. I told them I had a friend with a nail salon who was interested too, and they said they'd sell me two for £6,000 each. So, the concept of 'FiFi's Fabulous Fannies' was born – a franchise of vaginal tightening salons across the nation! What more could you ask for? Regulations, perhaps? The fact that I could do that, and not be stopped by anyone, is beyond comprehension because unqualified people playing around with your vagina and pelvic floor function is a recipe for disaster – but again, here we are.

For Vikram Talaulikar, the current landscape is unacceptable. He says these types of products should be taken off the market until they can prove that they aren't dangerous. 'Show me a randomised controlled trial [RCT]. That would be my answer to it, unless you've done a big RCT and shown me it's at least neutral and the study was not funded by you, and you're not manipulating results, you should not be bringing out a product at all.'

In many ways, we have things back to front, Weiss-Wolf says, 'Vaginal oestrogen could probably solve a lot of the problems these women are seeking treatment for including dryness and bladder issues, yet we still have out-of-date warnings that frighten people away from using those products even though we know they are safe for the vast majority of people. But we have virtually zero regulations on things that make outrageous claims and could potentially do considerable long-term harm.'

Femtech

But, this isn't the only problem that's keeping Weiss-Wolf awake at night – Femtech is too.

Don't be fooled into thinking it's a few geeky start-ups with great ideas waiting to blossom, the Femtech industry is huge. In 2021 the market was worth $51 billion and by 2030 it's expected to be worth $103 billion.[33] Why does that matter? Because many of them are making money off your health data and it's worth a lot. It's estimated the NHS data alone is worth £9.6 billion. Menopause data is a relatively new thing – there wasn't much of it about before but now we're sharing information on apps, Fitbits and online surveys like no tomorrow, and there are very few safeguards around its use.

'There's a lot of concern about digital safety such as the protection of privacy of your digital footprint. So, there are some reforms that matter here too to protect women as some of it can be outwardly dangerous, like period tracking,' Weiss-Wolf says.

How so, you ask? In today's pro-life, anti-abortion climate in the US, Weiss-Wolf is concerned that these types of apps could result in punishment or punitive actions being taken against women around reproductive decision-making.

Many of these apps or sites offer communities where women can gather and share their opinions or experiences with certain treatments or procedures. Michelle Griffin, gynaecologist and BBC columnist turned Femtech strategist, says that has its pluses. 'Women's health apps have revolutionised access to information, busted myths and built supportive communities. They can offer powerful insights into our health and wellbeing.' But, she says, 'some operate in a grey area, collecting deeply personal data with little transparency on how it's used. Women shouldn't have to trade privacy for progress and therefore the necessary data privacy requirements must be prioritised and baked into the development.'

It's a call backed by researchers at Newcastle University who say these types of tracking devices can pose significant security, privacy and safety issues for women using them, and that the intimate data collected by these Femtech systems was regularly processed and sold to third parties. They wrote: 'The findings have exposed a lack of research and guidelines for developing cyber-secure, privacy-preserving and safe products,' and they urged regulatory bodies to update and strengthen guidelines.[34]

One tracking app, Flo Health Inc, has already had an FTC complaint and a class action case brought against it in the United States for sharing data with companies like Facebook and Google[35] which could allow them to tailor ads to certain demographics. A class action has also been launched in Canada.[36] In a statement following the settlement of the FTC complaint in the US, Flo denied it has sold data to advertising departments and said it did not share anything that was identifiable such as names, dates of birth or addresses. Flo says it now doesn't share data without consent.[37]

Flo said:

> Allegations of events regarding user data between 2016 and 2019 led to an FTC investigation. It was alleged that Flo shared health information with third-party advertising companies without permission.
>
> This was not the case. Like many companies, Flo shared limited data with selected third-party companies to internally measure the performance of our app. None of this data contained our members' names, addresses, or birth dates. Nor did we share health information with the social media, advertising, or marketing departments of these third parties.
>
> Flo chose to stop sharing any information with these third parties in January 2021. At the same time, we agreed to settle the matter with the FTC. As a growing company, we made this decision to avoid the time and cost associated with litigation. It enabled us to instead focus our efforts on rolling out best-in-class security and privacy protections. Since then, Flo has become the only women's health app to be awarded dual International Organization for Standardization (ISO) certifications in privacy and security – widely recognized as the gold standard in the industry.
>
> We would like to make clear that this settlement was in no way an admission of wrongdoing. Flo continues to stand by its position. We have never, and will never, sell your data – nor will we share your health information with third parties for marketing purposes.

Flo may well be ahead of the pack then as a study in the UK found that 84 per cent of apps allowed the sharing of personal and sensitive health data beyond the developer's system with third parties. Some 68 per cent sold data for marketing, 40 per cent for research and 40 per cent for improving developer services of the app itself.[38] Dr Josie Hamper, an online digital health and trust researcher at the University of Oxford, has spent over a decade researching health app use and says women know their data is being sold.[39] 'Telling the users of tracking apps that their data is being shared in these ways generally won't surprise them. They know – or at least have some inkling – that their data is valuable beyond the app, and they know that this is tied to a much broader commercialisation of women's health and bodies. But the promise of improved health knowledge and "insights" keeps users interested – and invested – in their apps. The risk is that over time, this acceptance through continued use normalises poor privacy protections.'

Does it matter, you ask? You're menopausal so who cares if they know you're drowning in sweat at night or seeing a pelvic floor physio to help stop your bladder leakage? Health insurers might, Weiss-Wolf says: 'You might think it's benign that you're tracking all this information, but it's going into some big consumer database that health insurance companies can now somehow have the data they need to justify jacking up certain rates and premiums. So those are the things I think about when I think about the commercial market.'

They may also use it to add more exclusions to treatments or cover because you have a pre-existing condition. Employers might like this kind of data too – after all they know 'women of a certain age' are more likely to take days off due to our symptoms. And advertisers will love it because they know they can sell this group supplements, cooling sprays and absorbent underwear. (I'd prefer a plan for a pelvic floor physio – but we all know the former will be there first!)

One London-based company called Kaleidoscope, which helps start-ups overcome the challenges with data protection, says privacy is tough to navigate but the implications can be significant. Data privacy specialist Amy Ford told Femtech World: 'Not processing personal and sensitive health data in a safe and lawful way could lead to an infringement on the rights and freedoms of women. These could be loss of control over their personal data, discrimination and profiling, reputational damage, loss of privacy, limited access to services, loss of anonymity, exclusion and bias and even surveillance by authorities. Failure to protect users' data could cause irrevocable damage and life-altering changes to women and their families.'[40] Strong stuff.

The flip side though is that all this data could help close the gender data gap – but the challenge, Griffin says, is to handle it well. 'Closing the gender data gap is crucial, and women's health apps can play a key role in the solution. The wealth of real-world data from these apps could help researchers better understand conditions that have been historically underfunded, improve treatments, and potentially shape more inclusive healthcare policies. Often the real-world data can be the starting point to trigger a scientific research and clinical study which leads to essential findings and possible health treatments. But this has to be done correctly, ensuring that the relevant data is collected in the appropriate manner under comprehensive data consent, privacy and governance standards, stored securely and used properly.'

But bridging that gap might be harder than it seems. Even though the Femtech market is 'the next big thing', it too has its own misogyny with angel investors seemingly biased against projects looking at women's health. The McKinsey report looked at the market and found that there were eleven start-ups seeking funding for men's conditions including erectile dysfunction (ED) and eight start-ups looking for funding for endometriosis.[41] The men's projects secured $1.24 billion between 2019 and 2023 while the endometriosis ones attracted about a third of that amount, landing just $44 million. Yes, ED is quite common with one in five men experiencing it at some stage in their life, and it can be an indicator of an underlying heart condition. Endometriosis, on the other hand, is said to affect one in ten, but it's massively under-diagnosed and can take up 8–12 years to diagnosis, so the actual figure may be much higher. And we've seen the cost in terms of physical and mental pain, surgery and missed work.

The ED market is quite competitive with many drugs, like Viagra, already available, but there's very little except progesterone and pain killers that can help with endometriosis, so you'd think there would be a considerable opportunity there for the savvy investor – but that funding discrepancy suggests the appetite for funding women's health is limited. According to the *Women's Health Matters* report, that's a shame. Its analysis of the burden of over 350 health conditions shows 5 per cent are exclusive to women – like endometriosis – and 95 per cent of the others, which includes conditions like heart disease, affect women differently, and these present 'an immense opportunity for breakthroughs in research, innovation, and investment'.[42]

So, there are huge opportunities out there, but the trick will be making sure that the research delivers effective treatments, rather than those that are designed for profit over real patient benefit.

3

WHY IT MATTERS – YOUR FUTURE HEALTH

I'm interested in women's health because I'm a woman. I'd be a darn fool not to be on my own side.

– Maya Angelou

Around menopause and afterwards there are silent changes happening to our bodies that we may not notice but they can have a profound impact on our future health. These next few chapters will look at what the main changes are and what we can do about them to reduce our risk of poor health later in life.

And remember: the changes you make today can make a positive impact on your health span and your longevity, and it's never too late.

Enjoy!

7

What did I come in here?
The brain: dementia and mental health

If that title sounds familiar to you, fear not, because you are in fact in the right place. This chapter is on your brain, what we know so far about why you can't remember what you came here for or why you're feeling down, and what you can do about it.

There are so many comedy skits about conversations with menopausal women – you know, the ones where 'thingamajiggy is talking to that woman, you know her – what's her name? It'll come to me. She was in the film with the actor, you know the one, he looks like the other one. What's his name?' Those conversations. But when it's happening to you with familiar regularity, it's not quite so funny.

Like many women, when this started to happen to me I thought I was going mad, dementing, that I had early onset Alzheimer's disease – a rare form that affects women under the age of 65. A bit dramatic, you say? Not necessarily, when you consider my family history. My mother was diagnosed with this when she was 58 and she was dead a decade later. Her mother had some kind of early onset 'senile dementia', which is what they called it back in the late 1960s, and she, too, was dead in her 60s. So, you can imagine, every time I can't remember a word, where my glasses are (usually on the top of my head), where I put my keys, or what the hell I'm looking for in the fridge, I think, 'this is it, the beginning of the end'. It's like a sword of Damocles hanging over your head, always in the back of what you think is left of your mind.

I did chat to my doctor when it started, in early perimenopause. He told me it was probably stress related, and I do think it's worse when my stress levels are higher than usual. I had hoped it would go away then I started MHT a decade ago, but I still wander into rooms wondering what I came there for. Anyway, if this sounds like you – welcome to 'brain fog'. But it's not just forgetting words or where things are – it messes with many more things than that. It affects your concentration, your ability to multi-task – to just get stuff done! But if you think you're alone, take heart: studies show this brain fog is very common, affecting somewhere between 44–62 per cent of women.[1]

Unlike me, you probably don't have a history of early onset dementia in your family, but maybe you have a history of late-onset Alzheimer's disease, which happens after age 65 and affects about 20 per cent of women, or maybe Alzheimer's disease doesn't run in your family at all but you fear you may be the first to get it. Regardless, like me, you may worry that if you aren't dementing now, this brain fog could be a harbinger of things to come. So, when claims are made that taking MHT could perhaps prevent it, you want to believe them. Now, I'm not going to lie, I am secretly hoping that by taking it I may not end up following in the same steps as my mother and grandmother, and on paper the claim makes logical sense. It goes like this: what's good for the heart is good for the brain and we believe oestrogen is good for the heart – true. Oestrogen is anti-inflammatory and neuroprotective – true. So, replenishing declining oestrogen should, in theory, help prevent dementia. But, and it's a big but – at the moment we just don't know for sure if it does. The evidence is conflicting and we simply don't have enough of it.

BMS-accredited menopause specialist and pharmacist with a special interest in mental health, Kate Organ says, 'The fear of dementia is one of the most prominent concerns I hear from women in my menopause clinic. The media's attention to HRT being linked to a potential reduction in risk is therefore a glimmer of hope for many women, particularly if there is a family history of dementia. But HRT will not treat dementia and it's important to get the correct diagnosis so you can receive the correct care. I have certainly been asked on several occasions to prescribe HRT for women with quite prominent cognitive symptoms who are, or should be, being further assessed in memory clinics. Even family members of women who have received a dementia diagnosis have asked, as they're willing to try anything to ward off cognitive decline.'

Dr Sam Brown, a BMS-accredited menopause specialist with a special interest in mental health, understands the frustrations of the conflicting research, but says at this stage 'I would not start a woman on HRT if she described no symptoms at all related to menopause, but said she wanted to start HRT in order to prevent dementia. I do not think we have the evidence to do this, but this may change in the future.'

She, too, says she has many women who book in to to discuss their brain fog. 'They feel like they're almost certainly developing dementia and feel a sense of shame about how they are coping. They are also very worried about the future, particularly if they have a family history of dementia. Brain fog, along with irritability, is a very common reason for women to book in because these symptoms very much impact on their work, relationships and general functioning.

'The women I see in midlife have worked their way up the career ladder and are often at the top of their game in the field they are in. Then the rollercoaster of perimenopause comes along. As a result of this and the general overwhelm they often think about leaving work or going part-time as they have lost confidence in their own abilities. They often say that they can forget names, forget what they are saying mid-sentence or forget conversations hours after. They have multiple Post-it notes, lists and struggle to stay focused or on task. They forget conversations with partners and children, and can become the target of family jokes as a result of this.'

Organ says, 'One of the key clinical indicators of cognitive symptoms of the menopause is the presence of other menopausal symptoms. It is rare that women will present with cognitive symptoms alone. Brain fog symptoms will be transient and are generally not progressive in nature, they do not involve disorientation to time or spatial dysfunction, changes to behaviour like wandering or irritability, or affect ability to complete day-to-day tasks. Menopausal brain fog often improves when other menopausal symptoms which may impact on sleep such as night sweats, nocturia [having to get up to pee], and itching are treated.

'It is often such a relief when they realise that this is very common, related to the menopause and should, eventually, improve. Self-care, a good diet, reducing alcohol, a good sleep routine, reducing stress, regular aerobic exercise, mindfulness and HRT can all be helpful, and I can support them in finding what works best for them.'

So, why isn't MHT currently recommended as a way of preventing dementia? First, to make an enormous understatement – the brain is a hugely complex thing and, despite what we're told on social media, we don't know much about it in general, let alone what happens to it in menopause. But work is underway, and one scientist who has attracted a lot of attention recently is Dr Lisa Mosconi, an Associate Professor of Neuroscience in Neurology and Radiology at the Weill Cornell Medical College in New York and author of three books on the brain including *The Menopause Brain*.

Speaking on a podcast with the US-based patient advocacy group 'Let's Talk Menopause', Mosconi explained why she started to look at oestrogen in the brain as a way to explain the difference in the incidence of Alzheimer's between men and women.[2] She and her team were looking at a variety of factors that could account for women being twice as likely to get it and were asking if those changes started in midlife. They were looking at diet, lifestyle, cholesterol and triglycerides as causes, but it was a chance encounter with a woman who was having a hot flush during a cognitive test that sent her down the menopause route – could this be the missing link – the one thing that differs between men and women? This was her 'aha' moment back in 2014.

She and her colleagues mapped the brains of women who were at different reproductive stages and in 2021 released a study showing there were 'profound effects' on the way it functions when we hit perimenopause and beyond.[3] This does get a bit geeky in spots, but bear with me. They did PET scans on 161 cognitively healthy women aged 40–65. Some 42 per cent had the APOE4 gene – the one that's associated with a great risk of Alzheimer's, and 13 per cent of the perimenopausal group were on hormone therapy as were 32 per cent of the postmenopausal group.

The scans showed what the different regions of the brain were doing and what the brain looked like in pre-menopause, perimenopause and postmenopause. When they compared pre-menopausal brains to the perimenopausal brains they found that perimenopausal ones had less grey matter and less white matter in certain areas. Grey matter, again in certain areas of the brain, is crucial in information processing, memory and emotions. White matter has a role in sending information around the body but it is also important in the communication pathways between different parts of the brain, learning and problem solving. The team also looked at the way the brain used energy sources and noted that as oestrogen dipped in perimenopause the brain's metabolism system was working overtime to fuel itself and maintain its function. This suggested that it was resilient and adaptable.

When they looked at the postmenopause brains, most looked as though they had stabilised or showed an increase in grey matter in those regions again – so they had adapted, or 'recovered' for want of a better word. The researchers also found that the protein – beta amyloid ($A\beta$) – was more pronounced in women who carried the APOE4 gene which is associated with Alzheimer's disease (AD). These are, Mosconi says, 'red flags' for Alzheimer's. 'They're not a diagnosis of Alzheimer's, just a sign that your brain may be in danger of developing Alzheimer's later on in life.'[4] And the study hypothesised that 'while some women in our cohort might eventually develop AD, for others, $A\beta$ deposition could reflect accelerated biological aging due to hormonal declines instead. In fact, over 20 per cent of healthy elderly display moderate cerebral $A\beta$ burden and no dementia.'[5] And that's important because it's estimated that around a third of cases of Alzheimer's could be prevented through some very simple lifestyle changes – and we'll get to that.[6]

Then came a 2023 analysis of six randomised controlled trials involving 21,065 treated and 20,997 placebo participants and 45 observational studies with 768,866 patient cases and 5.5 million controls that Mosconi was a co-author on.[7] Now, these are big numbers! The analysis showed a potential 32 per cent reduction in cases of Alzheimer's and concluded that oestrogen therapy (not combined therapy – oestrogen and a progestogen) 'initiated during the critical window of the menopause transition may support neurological function and reduce the risk of future AD among eligible women'. But, it went on to note its own limitations saying: 'We recognize and emphasize the inherent limitations of relying largely on observational data and that stronger, randomized controlled trial evidence is needed to fortify these conclusions. Overall, these findings provide new insights on the association between HT use and AD incidence, and support renewed research interest in evaluating HT for the purpose of AD and dementia risk reduction.'

Why the caveat? Because observational studies may show an association but they don't show cause and effect. One of the large observational studies included in this analysis looked at the insurance records of around 380,000 Americans[8] and showed that those who took MHT had fewer cases of dementia but, even though it's a big number of people they looked at, they were mostly White (77 per cent), and by virtue of the fact that they could afford health insurance they were probably relatively well off, educated and employed, meaning it's not representative of the population in general. The authors listed their own limitations too including the limited length of time for follow-up, the age when people started therapy wasn't known, they couldn't account for changes in the types they took over time, how bad their symptoms were, or whether or not they had genes associated with Alzheimer's.

The study isn't without its critics too, who questioned the data they chose to include in their analysis.

Despite this, headlines started to appear like this one from CNN saying 'Sweet spot for HRT may reduce dementia risk by nearly a third, study says'.[9] And, as a result, another theory arose: even if you don't have menopause symptoms, you should be on MHT or your brain would be at risk. On social media people who couldn't take hormones because of cancer or weren't on MHT started to post about being 'left out' of the discussion or having 'FOMO' (fear of missing out) if they weren't taking oestrogen. I don't think I can count the number of people who've asked me 'should I take it? I don't have symptoms but now I'm worried I'll get dementia if I don't.'

Then in 2024, Mosconi and her team released another study that showed that the menopause transition was marked by a 'progressively higher density of estrogen receptors' on the brain cells, and this lasted well into these women's 60s.[10] This time they scanned the brains of 54 healthy women aged between 40–65 using a 'tracer' that binds to oestrogen receptors so you can see where they are. Eighteen women were pre-menopausal, 18 were perimenopausal and 18 were post-menopausal. What they found was the peri and post women's brains lit up in certain areas where there were many more receptors, and they interpreted this as 'a compensatory response to waning levels of available estrogen – as estrogen levels drop during the menopause transition, the cells express additional receptors to sop up as much estrogen as possible,' Mosconi said in a press release.[11] The study also found that the high receptor density in some of regions of the brain was associated with the 'patients' reports of menopause-related cognitive and mood symptoms'. They went on to suggest that this scanning technique could be a valuable tool for evaluating whether oestrogen therapy made any difference. In the press release Mosconi suggested that their finding 'hints that the "window of opportunity" for estrogen therapy may be greater than thought' while the study concluded it 'posited [the] "window of opportunity" for preventative strategies'.

Pulling that all together we've got functional brain changes, brain receptors that are literally screaming out for oestrogen that are matched to people who've self-reported cognitive issues and may have increased deposits of Alzheimer's-related plaques that are a 'red flag' for developing the disease later in life: surely the answer is replace the oestrogen to prevent these changes? Combine that with the fact that we know women who have Premature Ovarian Insufficiency, who go through menopause before the age of 40, are at higher risk of cognitive decline and Alzheimer's,[12] and that women are twice as likely to develop Alzheimer's than men – and you've got a very powerful argument that oestrogen prevents dementia.

So, it's easy to see how over time, somewhere, somehow, things started to get a little lost in translation. For example, what was 'hinted' as a theory for future research on the timing of preventative strategies was getting picked up in the media with headlines like this one from Oprah: 'How estrogen therapy could prevent dementia.'[13] A popular podcast from biohacking guru and entrepreneur Dave Asprey featuring a diet and science journalist, Max Lugavere, whose mother had early onset Alzheimer's and wasn't on MHT is another example. Asprey claimed the stigma around hormone replacement that saw women denied access was 'the biggest crime against women'[14] while Lugavere said the loss of oestrogen was like having the 'rug pulled out' from under women's feet. And then Dr Roberta Diaz Brinton from Arizona University, who was a co-author on the 380,000-strong insurance study, brought it home in *Science Daily*[15] with a widely quoted statement: 'The key is that hormone therapy is not a treatment, but it's keeping the brain and this whole system functioning, leading to prevention. It's not reversing disease; it's preventing disease by keeping the brain healthy.' But what wasn't more widely quoted was the other part of the sentence that theorised that 'with this study, we are gaining mechanistic knowledge. This reduction in risk for Alzheimer's disease, Parkinson's and dementia means these diseases share a common driver regulated by estrogen, and *if there are common drivers*, there can be common therapies.'

Possible common drivers aside – surely then all roads must lead to Rome, we must be missing a trick by not universally taking MHT to prevent dementia

It's a logic that Dr Pauline Maki understands well because she walked this path herself a couple of decades ago. She may not be a big name on social media but she's huge in the world of menopause and brain research. In fact, she is one of the world's most respected and award-winning researchers in this field. She works quietly behind the scenes to do the studies that form the guidelines that are the basis for evidence-based medical practice. She is a professor of psychiatry, psychology and gynaecology and obstetrics at the University of Illinois in Chicago. She is the one who discovered how hormone therapy affects the brain back in the late 1990s/early 2000s, and was looking at exactly the same thing way back then.

'I'll tell you, I was, quote, "a believer". I thought, "oh, universally, it looks as though the loss of oestrogen alters memory, it alters brain function and the like". But then the randomised trial data came out, and it wasn't just one study, it wasn't just two studies, it was four large-scale randomised trials that showed that in women without significant hot flashes, hormone therapy had no effect on them. None. Zero. Zip. So, I had to accept those data and say, you know what? I was wrong. I based it on the observational data. I thought it would have an effect, and it didn't,' she told me in an interview for the Menopause Research and Education Fund.

She says many of the benefits touted for taking oestrogen to prevent dementia have been cherry-picked from observational studies while the majority actually show 'it's exactly, and I mean exactly, the opposite. The four most recent large-scale observational studies have actually shown a significant increased risk of Alzheimer's disease in women who've used hormone therapy. And it doesn't matter what the formulation is, it doesn't matter what the route of administration is, it doesn't matter what oestrogen or progesterone you choose, the signal is there. So, I think there can be a selectivity, and when I see some of these "pro" oestrogen for cognition stances . . . I'll see them select data from those studies that isn't the data that was in the abstract of the original studies. It isn't the data that the people who wrote the papers thought was the most important. It's kind of like they go in and they select something that looks a little bit better. But I think we need to be as objective as possible when we make these decisions about what to recommend to women.'

Some of the studies she's referring to are:

- Finland: In a case-control study involving 84,000 women MHT was related to a 9 per cent increase in Alzheimer's cases for those taking oestrogen alone (ET) and a 17 per cent increase in those taking combined oestrogen and progestogen therapy (EPT).[16]
- UK: A study of 118,501 women showed overall a neutral result – no increased or decreased risk of dementia or Alzheimer's.[17] When it came to all cause dementia, oestrogen only for ten years or more was associated with a 15 per cent decreased risk among those younger than 80 years. For Alzheimer's, combined therapy yielded a different result with oestrogen and progestogen use for five to nine years associated with a 10 per cent increased risk of dementia. For more than ten years of use there was a 20 per cent increase. While the percentages sound large, it equates respectively to five and seven extra cases per 10,000 woman-years – so if 100 women used it for ten years there would be five or seven extra cases. The researchers said different progestogens carried different risks too.
- Denmark: A 2023 study looking at 5,589 cases of dementia and 55,890 age matched controls aged 50–60 years with no history of dementia or contraindications for use of menopausal hormone therapy.[18] They found MHT was positively associated with dementia and Alzheimer's but said, 'Further studies are warranted to determine whether these findings represent an actual effect of menopausal hormone therapy on dementia risk, or whether they reflect an underlying predisposition in women in need of these treatments.'

And it's that last sentence that is really important because there is an argument that those with severe and perhaps poorly controlled symptoms are more likely to take MHT in the first place and as such the figures are skewed to show that more people on hormone therapy develop dementia/Alzheimer's because they were at far higher risk in the first place.

The upshot

So, what are we looking at then? At the moment, it is at best a neutral effect depending on the type of MHT used and the length of time it's used for. But, what about that 2017 Women's Health Initiative study of 27,000 women, which showed there was a 26 per cent reduced risk of Alzheimer's disease in the women who took the oestrogen alone and a decrease in deaths from dementia and Alzheimer's, I hear you say? Maki says this was 'exciting news. Something prevented dementia.' And a 26 per cent reduced risk is not to be sneezed at – that's big! But the question is how do you translate this epidemiological study to your decision about treating a patient, or if you are a patient how do you decide it you should take it yourself? Is your own risk reduced by 26 per cent?

'The way that we do that is through the calculation of the number of women you would need to treat with hormone therapy to prevent one case of dementia, and if that number is low – if I only need to treat 10 women to prevent a case of dementia then that suggests, okay, maybe this should change medical practice,' Maki says. In this case however, 'you need to treat 2004 women to prevent one case of dementia . . . That means 2003 women took it without getting any benefit.' That's a lot of people to treat to avoid one case of Alzheimer's.

Dr Maki adds there are flaws in the logic too when it comes to menopause even being a risk factor and the much-touted statistic of women being twice as likely to develop dementia or Alzheimer's. The argument goes that the higher rate in women can't just be because women live longer as it's really only a couple of years now, so the only other difference between men and women is menopause and our loss of oestrogen. And yes, it is true that women are twice as likely as men to develop these conditions, but an interesting fact that's often not made clear is that up until our late '70s to early '80s our incidence rates are virtually equal.[19] And in women, dementia and Alzheimer's were both diagnosed about a year later than in their male counterparts – men were usually 80 or just under and women were just over at 81. To put that another way, men were developing it at about the same rate until around 80 and were being diagnosed at a slightly younger age than women. It's when we're over 80 that we take over.

'Let's look at a group of 70-year-old women,' Maki says. 'What percentage of them have been through this loss of oestrogen? One hundred per cent. And what proportion of those women will get demented? About 20 per cent. What proportion of men will? About 19 per cent. So really, is there this cause effect issue with the loss of oestrogen and Alzheimer's disease? It can't be that simple. The data just don't bear it out.'

The vulnerable brain

But something is clearly afoot so the next question is, who then are the vulnerable women?

'In my mind, it's the many, many, many women who've gone untreated for their menopause symptoms. I still adhere to the belief that we must increase the uptake of hormone therapy for symptomatic women, absolutely, 100 per cent agree with that, because I think it does protect their brain'. And perhaps this is where the two views intersect – not with the drop in oestrogen manifesting across the brain as the cause but the vasomotor symptoms it produces, the effects they have and how well they're treated. As Dr Maki explains, 'This is a critical issue. We do know that at minimum, women who have persistent hot flashes are at increased risk for cardiovascular events, cardiovascular disease and cognitive decline. What we don't know is whether or not that's causal.'

When it comes to cognition, however, we have 'a proof of concept that if you treat the hot flashes, memory improves. We know that because we did a randomised trial of a non-hormonal intervention called stellate ganglion blockade'– a procedure that involves injecting an anaesthetic into a specific location in the neck. 'The reason I used it is because it's not known to improve cognition generally, but it treats hot flashes. And we asked the question, if you took away the hot flashes does memory get better? And the good news is, it did show some evidence of cause and effect for the hot flashes and memory.'

Her theory is that vasomotor symptoms at night might be, in part, the biggest culprit because they disrupt sleep – and while we generally associate hot flushes at night with women waking in a pool of sweat, some women don't even know they're having them. During one of her trials Maki wore a sensor at night and was surprised to find she had three hot flushes that she absolutely had no idea about. Even though you may not notice them, they can still disrupt sleep and leave their mark on the brain. She says when you look at the brains of people with vasomotor symptoms they resemble those of people who have sleep apnoea, a condition where breathing stops repeatedly through the night, disturbing your deep restorative sleep (see Chapter 10). It's often characterised by loud snoring and gasping for air, so if your partner keeps waking you saying 'your snoring could wake the dead' – get it checked!

Maki says there are 'associations between stroke-like lesions in the brain called white matter hyperintensities and hot flashes, and that's exactly what you see with sleep apnoea, and it's exactly what you see with hypertension. And so, you take these multiple risk factors – let's say I have a little hypertension, I have a little sleep apnoea, and I have my hot flashes – well suddenly my female brain is very vulnerable.'

We know that 'women do feel better on hormone therapy, and I think their cognition may very well feel better, but it's probably because they're having fewer hot flashes, they're sleeping better, and maybe their mood is a little bit better because of all that'. But if they don't have vasomotor symptoms 'there's zero evidence to suggest it's beneficial' when it comes to dementia prevention.

There is perhaps some good news for preventing early onset dementia, she says, with the MIRAGE study showing there was a potential benefit for lowering the risk of developing dementia between the ages of 50 and 63.[20]

Both Maki and Mosconi have a family history of Alzheimer's too. My mother wasn't on MHT. She was a heavy smoker who never exercised – probably not since she was made to at school, although I do have a vague recollection of her going through a yoga phase in her 40s, but I can guarantee she had probably never even seen the door of gym let alone gone through one! She was well educated, an avid reader and ate well (always home cooked food and at least three different coloured veggies with every meal) but she was basically sedentary and overweight. When I was at university I remember her hot flushes – they were doozies. She literally turned purple and was drenched from head to toe within seconds, and she had a lot of them. She also, like Maggie Thatcher, never slept more than four or five hours and when she did sleep, boy did she snore. I always thought it was dad until I went into their room one night to wake him up because I couldn't sleep, only to find him with his eyes wide open while the windows shook. (He was a very patient man!) I look back now and wonder if MHT would have made a difference. I'll never know of course, but I have made lifestyle changes just in case. I stopped smoking just before I turned 40, I've always exercised and, up until COVID, had a healthy BMI (could do with losing a bit now), and I've cut back on the alcohol. I also eat very well (too much, but very well), with loads of fresh fruit and veggies, and oily fish at least three times a week for my omega-3 (which is said to be good for the brain). I also take a vitamin D supplement for my bones and because a deficiency has also been associated with dementia.

While we seem to be finding few points of agreement at the moment, one everyone agrees on is the importance of a healthy lifestyle, and it seems it's never been more important. In the US they are predicting that there will be a doubling of dementia cases by 2060 in women, with Black adults faring worst.[21] Currently the lifetime risk of dementia for women is approximately one in four, but researchers project this is going to more than double to 48 per cent by 2060.[22] For men the rate will jump from 12 per cent to 35 per cent – almost tripling. Now, this is us – this is our lifetime risk – and the driving factors are those that hit particularly hard at menopause: rising rates of obesity, diabetes and heart disease. But the good news is it's estimated that around 50 per cent of dementia cases can be avoided by paying attention to the modifiable risk factors – the things we can change. So, what are they? *The Lancet* has published a good long list:[23]

- Get your high blood pressure under control.
- Decrease your risk of diabetes (eat well with lots of fruit and veggies and less refined sugar – a Mediterranean-style diet is highly recommended).

- Try not to get a head injury.
- Stop smoking (I know this is easier said than done, but if I can do it with a pack-a-day habit for 25 years, you can!)
- Avoid air pollution (again easier said than done, but if you can't move, you could try an air purifier).
- Try to keep a healthy weight.
- Exercise regularly – they say at least 150 minutes a week. (Brisk walking, weights/resistance training are good options for brains, hearts and bones).
- If you have depression, make sure it's managed well.
- Cut down on alcohol.
- Get your hearing checked – if you're going deaf there's a tendency to isolate yourself and we don't want that because the next point is . . .
- Stay social. Join a community group or club, volunteer somewhere, see your friends and family.
- Keep your brain active – having a higher level of education is associated with a lower risk as you have more 'brain reserve' – but it's never too late to exercise the grey matter!

Some lists have added regular sight checks to this for the same reason as hearing, the risk of social isolation. In the future it's hoped that vascular changes could help predict some types of dementia too.[24] Prioritising sleep is another – so if vasomotor symptoms or sleep apnoea are ruining your sleep, get them sorted.

'I'd hate to see women not engaging in the things that we do know improve our brain health and make our brains more resilient to Alzheimer's disease, and instead, take a pill [patch or gel] that you know at best is neutral if they don't have symptoms. So, we need to be prescribing and engaging in the activities that really work. But I fear that women will check the box mentally and say, "Oh, I'm on hormones. I've already done the hard work for dementia" instead of doing what we know can make a difference.' And that would be a real shame.

What about my mood?

Low mood, anhedonia (a loss of interest in life), anxiety, panic attacks and depression-like symptoms are common around menopause. Studies show that depression around menopause affects about one-third of women aged 40–58 and in the UK MHT is recommended if the symptoms are new.[25] Other countries' guidelines don't say this – but should they?

The 2024 International Menopause Society conference in Melbourne set out to answer the question with a debate entitled: 'Should MHT be first line for treating perimenopausal depression?' In the affirmative corner, Melbourne's own Professor Jayashri Kulkarni, a psychiatrist from the Alfred and Monash University. Her opponent, Dr Maki. Between them they have almost 700 published papers on menopause and the brain. A show of audience hands at the start revealed the majority of delegates were supporters of Professor Kulkarni's position and that Maki had her work cut out for her.

Professor Kulkarni argued that the current definitions of depression were inadequate when it came to patients in perimenopause. She said they presented differently and the hint was in the name – a depression that's caused by perimenopause. 'This is a different beast. It's severe. It's a type of depression that many women, around perimenopause onset, describe,' she said. She added these women have no history of previous depression and they often describe a series of specific symptoms including irritability and sometimes rage, loss of confidence, paranoia, anxiety and panic attacks as well as body aches and pains, sleep disorders, weight gain and suicidal ideation. She argued that depression was a complicated thing and we were only now beginning to understand the role of hormones – specifically oestrogen, progesterone and testosterone, and how they affect the brain.

'In the old days, when everything was much more simple,' Kulkarni explained depression was thought to be low serotonin or low noradrenaline levels. 'So, we'll just give you this drug called an SSRI. It'll prop up the serotonin and everything will be roses.' And it 'worked in about 40 per cent of people, but it doesn't work very well in this group'. What did work, she said, was replacing lost oestrogen and there were studies to back that up.

But do they cut the mustard? Maki argued that unfortunately they don't. Yes, she agreed, there are studies that show oestrogen can improve depressive symptoms in some women, but they're limited.

'Let's look at the quality of the data,' she told the audience. 'We have 148 women participating in clinical trials to see if [the main form of oestrogen] estradiol is effective. A whole 148 women. Are we going to practise medicine based on 148 women? No, I don't think so. The follow-up period is limited to a maximum of 12 weeks. Is that sufficient? Questions remain about the best progestogen to use, because these trials did not include a progestin. So fewer than 150 people, no progesterone, 12 weeks of follow-up. Are you going to practise medicine on that?' Her answer: 'no'.

She went on to argue that studies showed the vast majority of women with depressive symptoms in perimenopause do have a previous history of depressive symptoms and that it's not the decline in estradiol that's the problem, but the fluctuations. She cited studies that showed MHT wasn't effective in treating depression in postmenopausal women and added that the number of women who are vulnerable to fluctuations in perimenopause and depression is somewhere between 3 per cent and 11 per cent – 'so it's relatively rare,' and then she posed the question 'how do you identify that person in a clinical setting?'

And this is a tricky one. Many women in the UK complain that they've been incorrectly prescribed antidepressants when they should have been given MHT. Some 30 per cent say they were given antidepressants and 80 per cent of them felt that was 'inappropriate' for the symptoms they were experiencing, according to an article in *The Independent*.[26] But for a second, put yourself in the GP's shoes. You've got a ten-minute consultation. You tell the doctor you're not coping, you can't concentrate, you've lost interest in life, nothing makes you happy anymore, you can't sleep and sometimes you think you just don't want to be here anymore. Have you thought about committing suicide? Sometimes. We know that women's suicide rates rise between the ages of 45 and 54, according to Office for National Statistics (ONS) data on women in England and Wales, and while they have gone down steadily since the 1980s from 13.3/100,000 women to 7.5/100,000 in 2023, this age group – which coincides with most people's menopause – seems to be a time of higher risk.[27] Critics of this argument will say this is a crunch time for women on many fronts – teenage children, ageing and ill parents, pressures of work and finances – so something's gotta give!

But back to the consulting room – in that ten minutes you've mentioned a bunch of 'red flags' for depression, including suicidal ideation, so you could forgive your GP reaching for the prescription pad and thinking that antidepressants may be the first answer, because, you sound like you're at risk. As Maki explains: 'It's too difficult.' How do you in a time-pressured clinical setting determine which women have true clinical depression versus the one who has hormonal related depression – it's not easy and it's risky. 'Depression is too serious of an issue to get wrong,' she said.

'The World Health Organization reported that depressive and anxiety disorders were among the top 10 leading causes of disability worldwide for females, but not for males, and the global burden of disease in males and females is considerably greater in women. And what's the most severe outcome of depression – suicide. We need to use the evidence base for treating depression the way that we would for other aspects of menopause,' Maki said. 'So, is oestrogen a first-line therapy for perimenopausal women? No,' she argued, 'though it can be a very good thing to have in the toolbox for some.'

Did the audience agree? Had she changed their minds? A show of hands showed it was a close call but some in the audience were undecided. What there was agreement on was that there was a need for more research and that both SSRIs and MHT can often be used hand in hand.

Where does all that leave you – the person with the 'lived experience'?

As we know, many women have told numerous inquiries that they felt they weren't listened to, that they were 'fobbed off' with antidepressants, but when they finally got MHT their symptoms disappeared and they were back to their old selves again, a cloud lifted, sometimes within days.

But how do you know if that's you, or if you need antidepressants, or even both?

Australian GP Dr Ginni Mansberg says there are 'clues that might point it in one direction or the other. One of those is if a woman has a history of what is very suggestive of hormonal mood imbalance. So, the kinds of things that would make me sit up and take notice is a history suggestive of Premenstrual Dysphoric Disorder (PMDD), and often they don't know that it was PMDD. They always just thought that they had severe PMS. Another is women who had postnatal depression. Then there are those women who tell you that they always went psycho on the pill, these were women who were intolerant of synthetic progestins. Those women – my ears are pricked that this person could have what is more likely to be a hormonal component to their depression.

'The second thing is the characteristics of the actual depression. What we tend to see is less of is what we call anhedonia and sadness, but a lot of anxiety, with panic, people bursting into tears where they were not expecting it. These women often become quite socially phobic, so they avoid friends or don't answer text messages. They get quite anxious at the thought of a work event and make excuses not to go. They often describe flying off the handle and losing it and their husband and children tend to cop it. Often, they'll rally for work, but sometimes they say, "I don't even know what I'm doing at work. I'm just being awful and I'm so embarrassed." Those kinds of raging moments, they're really typical. And there's a slight paranoia – not hearing voices, not psychosis, but it's just taking things the wrong way, being overly sensitive. That kind of thing is really suggestive.'

The third thing, she says, is when all of this it comes on with other menopause symptoms like vasomotor symptoms, brain fog and insomnia. 'We don't have really good head-to-head trials of HRT versus antidepressants, and I think that they're coming, but I think there's a general consensus that antidepressants are less effective in this cohort of women.'

Kate Organ says about 5 per cent of her patients have suicidal ideation or thoughts of self-harm. 'For those women the addition of a conventional antidepressant can be helpful and needed in some cases to reduce suicidal risk and improve quality of life. This is a case-by-case situation. In my experience low doses are often adequate as an adjunct to HRT and can often be withdrawn over a relatively shorter timeframe compared to conventional treatment without HRT once hormones have been adequately stabilised at effective doses.'

Dr Mansberg agrees. It's not always black and white and there's no shame in that. 'I describe taking antidepressants as having a fling.

You're not marrying them, it's just a fling. And if you do end up doing this, that means you are somebody who wants your mental health to be better. Here's what it doesn't mean: It does not mean that you're a failure. It does not mean that you have not given anything else a go, that you're taking the easy way out. It does not mean that you're now on these medications forever. It means that you're going to have a short fling with something to make your life and the life of those around you better, and that's all it means, nothing else.'

If you are on one or the other, and you find it isn't making any difference then go back to your GP and discuss your options. What is important is that you get the right treatment for you and you may benefit from both.

Another thing that could help, Dr Brown says, is Cognitive Behavioural Therapy (CBT) especially if it's hormone-based depression. This is not sitting on a couch revisiting past trauma, it's a technique that trains you to think differently about any given situation and challenge the negative thoughts. I have done this for anxiety and its hugely helpful – a life skill. The current NICE guidelines say:[28]

> Consider CBT as an option for people who have depressive symptoms (not meeting the criteria for a diagnosis of depression) in association with vasomotor symptoms:
>
> * in addition to other management options or
> * for people for whom other options are contraindicated or
> * for those who prefer not to try other options.

Mansberg also suggests taking a look at the work of Kristin Neff, a psychologist who works on self-compassion. We are often kind to others but don't show ourselves the same kindness. This is not just 'mental masturbation' as she eloquently puts it – it's an investment in you, your brain and your family. And, she says there have been studies that show that it could even improve your vascular health – so it's an investment in your future health too![29]

Organ adds, the other important thing is lifestyle. Eating well, not drinking too much, reducing stress and getting regular exercise, making sure you sleep well, and having good social support – these are all vital. And, whether it's hot flushes, problems with cognition or mood – don't leave it untreated. There is help out there, and you are not alone.

8

Blood and bone, and your cardiometabolic health

Bones have secrets. Long after we're gone they can tell stories about our lives, or at least the way we led them. Some bones, like the pelvis and the forehead, can reveal what gender you were and the shape of the cranium may indicate ethnicity. Others, like the long bones in the arms and legs, can reveal if you were regularly active or sedentary and what kind or diet you had. And of course, they can show diseases like arthritis and osteoporosis. This was one of the things I found most interesting in studying anatomy – looking at the rough marks on the long bones from the thigh or calves and wondering what type of life this person had. Did all those lumps and bumps where the muscles and tendons attached mean they did a physically active job, were they athletic? If the bones were smooth and thin, were they an office worker or from a wealthy background and spent all day lazing on a chaise longue? But as fascinating as bones are in death, they're even more interesting in life, even though we tend to take them for granted.

We have 206 long, short, round and flat bones in our bodies that hold us up, move us around, protect our internal organs, help us breathe and maintain electrolyte or essential mineral levels like calcium and phosphorus in our bodies. While we used to think they were kind of boring, nothing could be further from the truth. Bones are constantly remodelling themselves – a process that's regulated by hormones. But over the past few years researchers have discovered that bones, especially the long ones like those in your arms and legs, may themselves play important roles in terms of releasing hormones that affect our metabolism. This is new and exciting stuff because they think they could influence in the way we use energy, insulin sensitivity, and even how much we eat and how we store fat. As this field develops, researchers hope these findings could result in new ways to diagnose, treat and even prevent obesity and metabolic diseases like diabetes, as well as conditions like osteoporosis.[1]

Why am I mentioning this in a book about menopause? Because around menopause our bones start to rapidly lose what's known as bone mineral density (BMD) with declining oestrogen levels driving the process. In a talk on preventing and treating osteoporosis given to the International Menopause Society (IMS), Professor Mike McClung, founding director of the Oregon Osteoporosis Center and global expert in bone health, explained that we reach peak bone mineral density in our late teens or early 20s. From then on it declines slowly – but when we hit the latter part of perimenopause, bone loss accelerates and we can lose up to 20 per cent of our BMD in the two or so years before menopause and the first few years after it. McClung, who worked on the development of the FRAX score that predicts the risk of a fragility fracture, believes we have to do more to identify the women who are entering this period with already lower than average BMD as they are at risk of developing osteoporosis by their mid-60s – a good 20 years early than those who have a average or good bone density. After that, the rate of loss slows again.[2]

If we lose too much bone density we may be at risk of developing osteopenia (lower bone mineral density) that may develop into osteoporosis, a condition where the bone mineral density is well below average and there is an increased risk of what's called a fragility fracture – that is, a fracture caused by things like falling over from a standing height, coughing or even lifting something.

Our blood work starts to change too. Our 'bad' cholesterol and triglyceride levels go up putting us at greater risk of heart disease and type 2 diabetes, and that in turn raises our risk of developing metabolic syndrome, a collection of health problems including central obesity, high blood pressure, high blood sugar, raised levels of the 'bad' cholesterol – the LDL, and high triglycerides. According to Professor Nanette Santoro, an obstetrician, gynaecologist, reproductive endocrinologist and infertility expert who also gave a talk to the IMS in early 2025, this is the time when plaques starts to accumulate in our carotid artery, our arteries become stiffer, and these changes continue after menopause, albeit at a slower pace. And if that weren't enough, that central obesity, or fattening around the middle, brings with it not just more subcutaneous fat (the fact that sits under the skin), it has the added bonus of delivering more visceral fat as well. This type of fat gathers around our internal organs and further increases our risk of heart disease. Her analysis shows that at menopause our risk of cardiometabolic diseases – heart disease, stroke, diabetes and obesity are around 10 per cent. Six years after menopause, it's 25 per cent. That's a big jump and menopause clearly plays a role.

How are those changes connected with bones? Bones make up 15 per cent of our body weight and they are constantly breaking down and rebuilding themselves, which means that we literally replace our entire skeleton every ten years or so. But this process releases minerals like calcium and phosphorus into the blood stream as well as a hormone called osteocalcin. Now this hormone, it's thought, could be integral to the way we burn energy and – wait for it – brain function, too.[3] Much more research is needed but some studies have shown that lower levels are associated with worse cognitive function in terms of memory and learning – in mice at least.[4,5] Now, we are not mice, but as research continues and links strengthen between the health of our bones and the hormones that can positively affect our heart, brain and metabolic health, keeping them in tip-top shape becomes even more important.

UK-based GP and menopause expert Dr Reem Al-Shaikh loves bones. She explains: 'They don't just hold us up and perform a bit of scaffolding, but they basically are part of our mineral storage. They're part of our hormone balance. They're part of our balance of calcium and vitamin D and phosphorus, and these are all minerals in our bloodstream that are really, really important to maintain good health. Our bones are what I would describe as very metabolically active.' She says the bone remodelling process looks a bit like this: 'There's a type of cell called an osteoblast and these are building block cells. They build bone. And then we've got the osteoclasts, which are the cells that breaks down bone and remodel them and these two guys need to work in harmony with each other all the time. And then we have a few osteocytes, and they're the overseers. They're making sure the bone matrix is good and strong. They're like the head teacher in a school – they've got the experience of how to get these other guys to play nicely.

'Now, the osteoblasts do something kind of cool – they produce hormones and one of the most important ones is osteocalcin. It can have an effect on multiple parts of our body including our pancreas, which is where insulin is made. It can actually stimulate the pancreas to make the insulin hormone. And that's really important because insulin is part of our glucose or sugar metabolism and our glucose balance is really important. It works well when we're sensitive to it.' If, we're not, or you have low insulin sensitivity, or insulin resistance as it's also called, you will need to produce more insulin to break those sugars down.[6]

Basically, what's happening is this: the food we eat is broken down into glucose and stored in muscle and fat for when we need it. Insulin, produced by the pancreas, is what carries the glucose out of the bloodstream and into those cells. If we eat too many sugary foods too often the pancreas will produce more insulin, but the fat and muscle cells start to ignore it, effectively stopping it from disposing of the excess glucose in the blood. As a result, our blood sugar levels begin to rise. Over time that can lead to type 2 diabetes.

'Imagine it was raining every single day,' Dr Al-Shaikh says. 'Eventually you'd stop wearing your boots, you'd stop carrying an umbrella, and you'd just say, "Whatever, I'm going to get wet." This is what happens when we've got too much insulin. Your body just goes, "Ah, let's just ignore it." And then suddenly we're starting to get metabolic problems, type 2 diabetes and visceral fat, which is not good. It's the nasty fat that encases organs and can cause problems like heart disease and fatty liver disease, so all these problems start to happen. But if we have a hormone that's basically making our cells, our muscles, more sensitive to insulin and improving the way we manage insulin, we can see how it could have quite a big effect on preventing some of these problems.'

So, osteocalcin is good at helping us manage blood sugars, but that's not all it can do. It plays a role in the production of another hero hormone called adiponectin, which can help reduce triglyceride levels. Triglycerides are a type of lipid or fat made from the foods we eat. Like blood sugar they are stored in fat cells and released when we need extra energy. Again, if our levels of these are too high it increases our risk of coronary heart disease. Dr Al-Shaikh says adiponectin is anti-inflammatory, and 'it can also improve our sensitivity to insulin, and it also improves the way we use our fat stores and the way we use energy, the way our muscles work. So again, you're starting to see how if you've got really strong bones, without even realising it, you're actually going to have really healthy bodily functions, and you may even burn fat better. So, it's just a kind of a wild idea that I want people to start really thinking about – that actually building bone strength could do more than just make stronger bones.'

Some studies have shown that people with metabolic syndrome have lower osteocalcin levels.[7] This doesn't mean that low osteocalcin levels cause metabolic syndrome or vice versa, but is pointing out the complex relationship between our bones and hormones.

Al-Shaikh's mantra is 'get strong, not skinny' – and this is why we need to pay extra attention to them as we head toward menopause and start to lose that BMD rapidly. We know that around 50 per cent of women over the age of 50 will end up having a fragility fracture and our risk increases with age. According to a WHO risk assessment, around one in ten women aged 60, one in five women aged 70, two in five women aged 80, and six in ten women aged 90 will have osteoporosis, and in 2007 it was estimated to affect more than 200 million women across the globe.[8] Its potential precursor, osteopenia (I say 'potential' because not all of those who have osteopenia will develop osteoporosis but it's a great warning bell) affects 54 per cent of postmenopausal women in the US and an additional 30 per cent are osteoporotic. By 80, these flip in favour of osteoporosis with 70 per cent osteoporotic and 27 per cent classed as osteopenic.[9]

And if you're thinking, 'meh, it's only really old people and a broken bone isn't that serious' – think again. An Australian study shows there was a considerable number of fragility fractures in woman aged 40–65. It found that between 1990 and 2012, 99,399 women with a mean age of 56.1 years had BMD tests. Of them, 52.5 per cent had normal results, 34.0 per cent were osteopenic and 13.5 per cent had osteporosis. Some 6,540 fragility fractures were reported with 66.8 per cent of them in women under the age of 65.[10]

And these come at significant cost. In 2025 it's estimated that 3 million people will have a fragility fracture in the US and around 13.5 million across the globe. Some 500 million people will have osteoporosis, mostly women, and the impact is huge, with direct costs to the health system in excess of $25 billion[11] in the US and $400 billion globally. To put that into perspective, fragility fractures account for around 3 per cent of healthcare costs and that is expected to double by 2050.[12]

In the EU the financial burden of fragility fractures is higher than some other common noncommunicable diseases. For example, osteoporosis costs were €37.4 billion in 2015, almost double the cost of coronary heart disease at €19 billion and the €20 billion spent on stroke, according to the International Osteoporosis Foundation.[13] In addition, fragility fractures significantly decrease quality of life and are one of the leading reasons why we lose independence and end up in care facilities. And, they can be fatal. Yes, fatal. Some 15–36 per cent of people who have surgery for a hip fracture will die within 12 months of that procedure.[14] You don't want to go there if you can avoid it – and neither does London-based GP Dr Elise Dallas.

Doctors get osteopenia too

Dr Dallas's mother recently fractured some bones in her thoracic spine coughing – yes, coughing. Her mother, now in her late 70s, has osteoporosis, was a smoker in days gone by and wasn't a great one for exercise, preferring 'skinny over strong' – as they did back in the 1970s and 80s. For most of her life she was a light, smaller-framed person at around 5 feet, and being small and light is a risk factor in itself. And, Elise says, she was on HRT but not for long – she was one of the many who flushed it down the toilet when the ill-fated WHI study came out back in 2002.

So, 48-year-old Dr Dallas did some maths and calculated that she'd probably lost about 8 per cent of bone density since her 20s. Then if you add the possible loss of another 20 per cent that she could be facing, she could end up losing around 28 per cent or almost a third of her bone mass. So, even though she does exercise, is on HRT, eats well and doesn't smoke or drink much alcohol, she decided to take herself off for a DEXA scan – a very low dose x-ray that gives you an indication of your bone mineral density. Your result is rated against that of a 30-year-old to give you a score of how far you are away from the peak. Her results came back with a score of –1, showing she was borderline osteopenic. (A score of above –1 is considered normal, –1 to –2.5 indicates osteopenia and below –2.5 may indicate osteoporosis.) She was shocked, but also in a strange way relieved, she says, 'because if I hadn't been doing all the good things, then I'd be in a far worse position'. Osteopenia can't be 'cured', so to speak, but it can be slowed, stopped or even reversed, and taking action can prevent it from developing into osteoporosis. Unsurprisingly, Dr Dallas isn't taking this lying down, she's upping her bone preservation game with a host of things.

Some of the things she's doing are:

- increasing weight and resistance training, including things like skipping. She says the LIFTMOR trial, which looked at two groups of post-menopausal women with a bone mineral density of <–1, found that those who underwent two training sessions a week for eight months of supervised high intensity resistance training outperformed those who undertook a home-based low intensity programme when it came to BMD improvements. So, she's hitting the gym.[15]

- making sure she has enough calcium in her diet – around 1,000–1,200mg/day is advised, so she's adding more green leafy vegetables, legumes, yoghurt and kefir.

- making sure she has enough vitamin D – she says around 800–1,000IU/day should be enough unless you have a diagnosed deficiency. She adds K2 and magnesium.

- looking out for her balance and posture. Balance is important as it can prevent you from falling and having good posture helps ensure your weight is distributed properly across your joints, so reducing the joint wear and tear. To that end she's adding in Reformer Pilates.

- prioritising her sleep. Night time is an important time in the bone remodelling process, so trying to get seven to eight hours of quality sleep is important.

- working on stress reduction as she says high cortisol levels can impact on the bone remodelling process too.

- making sure she has enough protein in her diet. She says 1–1.2gms of protein/kg of body weight is a good guide. There are various protein calculators you can use online to help you work out how much you need but depending on your age, weight and activity requirements somewhere between 45–65gms is a guide. Good sources of protein include lean meats, oily fish (especially those with the bones you can eat like sardines), eggs, soya, tofu and tempeh, peas and edamame beans, yoghurt and milk, and nuts and seeds.

Many people recommend a weighted vest but Dr Dallas warns they may not be suitable for all if you have previous injuries. She also says there's variable evidence on collagen supplements and bone density but if you can afford it, there's no harm in trying.

What are the risk factors for osteoporosis?

The International Osteoporosis Foundation has split them into things you can change (modifiable) and can't change (unmodifiable).[16]
The unmodifiable risk factors are:

- Your age – your risk increases with age
- Your gender – women are more likely to develop osteoporosis than men
- Your family history – you are at greater risk if your parents had osteoporosis or a broken hip
- You've had a previous fracture
- You've been through early menopause, menopause or POI.

The modifiable risk factors are:

- Excessive alcohol intake – drinking more than 2 units of alcohol per day increases the risk of fracture (some countries, such as the UK, say 3 units a day)
- Smoking – smokers have almost double the risk of hip fracture compared to risk in non-smokers
- Low Body Mass Index – being underweight with a BMI below 19 is a risk factor
- Poor nutrition
- Vitamin D deficiency
- Eating disorders like anorexia or bulimia can result in extreme weight loss, and if they cause menstruation to stop, this is a risk factor
- Being sedentary
- Low dietary calcium intake

- Frequent falls – people who have a tendency to fall are at higher risk of fracture, which may sound obvious, but it's why balance and strength exercise are so important.

Medications

Certain medications have side effects that are linked to osteoporosis or increased fracture risk. These include:

- Long-term glucocorticoid therapy – these medications (e.g. prednisone) are often used to treat arthritis or asthma; using glucocorticoids for three months or more places you at higher risk of fracture
- Proton pump inhibitors – these are used to treat reflux
- Certain medications to treat diabetes
- Certain antidepressants, anxiolytics, sedatives and neuroleptics
- Certain immunosuppressants (calmodulin/calcineurin phosphatase inhibitors)
- Thyroid hormone treatment (L-Thyroxine)
- Aromatase inhibitors (used to treat breast cancer)
- Certain chemotherapy agents
- Certain antipsychotics
- Certain anticonvulsants, anti-epileptics
- Anti-coagulants.

Speak to your doctor about the best way to preserve your bones if you are on these, or if there are alternatives.

Certain diseases

Some diseases may weaken bones and increase the risk of osteoporosis and fractures including:

- Rheumatoid arthritis (a major and common risk factor)
- Nutritional/gastrointestinal problems (lactose intolerance, Crohn's, inflammatory bowel, coeliac disease, etc.) which may affect absorption of nutrients
- Chronic obstructive pulmonary disease (COPD) and asthma
- Endocrine disorders including hypogonadal states, diabetes, Cushing's syndrome, hyperparathyroidism, Turner/Klinefelter syndrome, amenorrhea, etc.

- Immobility
- Chronic kidney disease
- HIV/AIDS
- Cancers (including prostate and breast cancer)
- Haematological (blood) disorders
- Dementia.

Again, if you have these, speak to your doctor about the best ways to help keep your bones healthy.

Endocrinology professor Annice Mukherjee has another to add to the list – restricted diets like very low-calorie diets, veganism, dairy-free or a diet that includes a lot of ultra-processed foods. 'If you're on any sort of restrictive or unbalanced diet, you have to make sure you get enough calcium, vitamin D and other micronutrients.' She recommends consulting a dietician.

If you don't know your family history, but you remember your parents or grandparents getting shorter and stooping, there's a good chance you have a genetic predisposition to osteoporosis. Dr Al-Shaikh says we've normalised the 'little old lady' but she is a walking example of exactly what we want to avoid.

Should you start MHT to prevent osteoporosis?

If you have gone through menopause before the age of 40 and there are no contraindications to MHT you should be on it anyway because we know you are at higher risk of osteoporosis. For other people without menopause symptoms it is not currently recommended as a way to prevent future bone loss. Some are arguing that this should change if you have specific risk factors. If you already have osteopenia or osteoporosis the Royal Osteoporosis Society says MHT 'can help to prevent bone loss and reduce your risk of developing osteoporosis and of breaking bones. If you already have osteoporosis or a high risk of breaking bones, HRT can help to strengthen your bones and make fractures less likely.'[17] Does that mean a healthy person who went through menopause at the average age, who has no menopause symptoms and has a normal bone density should take it to prevent future bones loss – at the moment the answer is no. But if you are on the road towards osteoporosis, that's a different story.

Professors Susan Davis and Annice Mukherjee have looked at the data on MHT and say the benefits are clear. 'A meta-analysis of RCTs [randomised control trials] assessing fracture risk in women using oral and transdermal estrogens (with or without the addition of a progestogen) reported a 20% to 37% reduced risk of hip, vertebral, and total fracture.' They said the effects are more pronounced in women under 60 using MHT, and that the protective effect wanes if the treatment is stopped, but it doesn't make the risk fracture worse. When it comes to treating osteoporosis, they argue MHT may be preferable in midlife women to some of the other treatments for osteoporosis. They wrote that while MHT was recognised in the guidelines as a treatment for postmenopausal osteoporosis it 'should be considered as a first option for bone protection in women with early or natural menopause over antiresorptive or osteoanabolic therapies, to delay the need for bone-specific therapy use'.[18] They added it was safe to continue it long term if the benefits continued to outweigh the risks.[19]

Should you have a DEXA scan?

If you think you are at risk and could benefit from having a DEXA scan to see what your score is, Dr Dallas recommends having a chat with your doctor about your risk factors and perhaps doing a FRAX test and taking that with you. You can find these online. These are some of the things the NHS says make you an eligible candidate for a DEXA – 'if you:

- are over 50 with a risk of developing osteoporosis
- are under 50 with other risk factors, such as smoking or a previous broken bone[20]
- have had a broken bone after a minor fall or injury
- have a health condition, such as arthritis, that can lead to low bone density
- have been taking medicines called oral glucocorticoids for three months or more – glucocorticoids are used to treat inflammation, but can also cause weakened bones

- are a woman who has had an early menopause, or you had your ovaries removed at a young age (before 45) and have not had hormone replacement therapy (HRT)
- are a postmenopausal woman and you smoke or drink heavily, have a family history of hip fractures, or a body mass index (BMI) of less than 21
- are a woman and have had large gaps between periods (more than a year).'[21]

Dr Al-Shaikh says the DEXA scan is the gold standard test for assessing your bone strength and ultimately fracture risk. Other tests are starting to come on the market that claim to assess your risk via your urine, fingernail clippings or ultrasound, but the DEXA is the one to go for – don't waste your money on the rest, she says.

And if you get a poor DEXA result it doesn't mean it's the end of the road, Dr Mukherjee says. 'At 60, if you sit on a chair and watch the television, don't do weight bearing exercise, lift any weights and have a poor diet you will likely be very frail when you're 80 or 90. But we know from thousands of people who are lifting weights in old age that you can prevent frailty through lifestyle. There is no drug that can compare. And I've got plenty of women on HRT who have other risk factors where HRT alone doesn't get their bones back to where it needs to be. Strength training, having enough calcium, vitamin D, not smoking, not drinking excessively, and addressing your stress are all crucial.'

Our cardiometabolic health

We don't often think of just how intertwined our heart health is with the rest of the body – but it really is, and it's taking a beating, says Mukherjee. In fact, 'it's deteriorating in pandemic proportions, with the rate of obesity and type 2 diabetes across the world rising'. These increase our risk of developing cardiovascular disease and dementia. In the UK the biggest killer is dementia/Alzheimer's disease, then heart disease, then cerebrovascular diseases like strokes.[22]

And when menopause hits, it creates a perfect storm which sees our risks rise rapidly. Studies show that postmenopausal women have a two-to-six-fold greater incidence of cardiovascular disease than their premenopausal counterparts up to the age of 54,[23] and by the time we've reached our mid to late 60s we've caught up with men in terms of incidence, and in our 80s more of us have cardiovascular disease than men.[24] We are also less likely to be diagnosed with a heart attack when we turn up at a hospital, we will wait longer for a diagnosis (on average 11–15 minutes depending on which study you look at), and if we are diagnosed we are less likely to be offered treatment to unblock an artery.[25] And even if we are, we're almost four times as likely to die within the next 30 days than a man (11.3 per cent compared to 3 per cent of men) and at five years afterwards, one-third of us (34.2 per cent) will have died in comparison to 19.8 per cent of men.[26] So, that's fun.

So, why do we get treated differently and have worse outcomes as a result?

It's often said women present with symptoms that may confuse doctors and lead to slower diagnosis or incorrect treatments. When we think of heart attacks we generally think of chest-clutching pain or pressure, left arm pain, back pain and maybe jaw pain, but women may also have things like tiredness, dizziness, nausea, vomiting, sweating, sleep disturbances, coughing and wheezing, reflux, and even anxiety. Traditionally these were referred to as 'atypical' symptoms but there are growing calls[27] to say goodbye to that terminology for a couple of reasons:

1 The primary symptom in women is still chest pain.
2 Using the word 'atypical' could suggest to those who are diagnosing you that the causes are not cardiac (heart-related), which can lead to delays or misdiagnosis.

And the British Heart Foundation agrees, saying women do have the traditional symptoms too.[28] So, the message is, focus on the heart.

But, there's another reason too. While the most common type of heart attack in both men and women involves a blockage of the larger blood vessels that supply the heart, women like to keep things interesting by throwing in a few variations.

Now, these may sound like fancy holiday destinations but a trip to INOCA, ANOCA or MINOCA, probably isn't one you want to take. They are in fact three different types of heart conditions that primarily affect women and may provide another reason for why we are treated later and differently.

Unlike blockages of major arteries, which are pretty easy to see on a standard angiogram, this trio are more difficult to see and affect the tiny, microvessels or the blood vessel walls themselves.

INOCA stands for Ischaemia with Non-Obstructive Coronary Arteries, and ANOCA is Angina with Non-Obstructive Coronary Arteries. Ischaemia means blood flow is constricted and angina is chest pain. MINOCA is Myocardial Infarction (or heart attack) with Non-Obstructive Coronary Arteries.

INOCA causes chest pain that can occur at rest or while exercising. There are two types – one that affects a significant portion of the small blood vessels that supply the heart muscle and another that causes a spasm in certain arteries which restricts the blood supply. To diagnose it they need to perform what's known as a functional coronary angiogram that tests for microvascular dysfunction and spasms. Around 40 per cent of all patients presenting with heart pain have these conditions but around 50–70 per cent are women.[29]

MINOCA, you'd think, would be the end stage of the other two – a heart attack after blood supply problems, but it can happen independently and is often caused by a disruption of plaques in blood vessels. It affects women more often than men and again, outcomes can be worse. In fact it's five times more common in women, accounting for around 10 per cent of our heart attacks[30] with some studies showing a range of 6–14 per cent.[31]

Another heart condition that affects women more than men is SCAD – Spontaneous Coronary Artery Dissection. Some 87 per cent of those who present with this are women. This unpleasant sounding thing is essentially a swelling of the layers in the heart arteries that leads to reduced blood flow and a heart attack. If you look closely on an angiogram it can be diagnosed by the line it causes in the artery wall. It tends to affect women in their 40s to mid-50s and strangely, they often don't have a lot of risk factors like high cholesterol or high blood pressure. That said, a big risk factor is being pregnant or the post-partum period as well as other vascular disorders, fibromuscular dysplasia and auto immune conditions such as SLE, and a history of migraines.

The last one that affects women more than men is 'broken heart syndrome' or Takotsubo cardiomyopathy. It makes up 1–2 per cent of heart conditions but more than 80 per cent of people who have this are women and they are often postmenopausal.[32]

Luckily, it's often reversible. It affects the left ventricle of the heart and is often triggered by acute emotional or physical stress. The symptoms are similar to a heart attack with chest pain, as well as shortness of breath or fainting.

It is diagnosed with a type of angiogram called an LV angiogram which will show a 'Takotsubo' – a ballooning of the left ventricle that looks like a Japanese crab pot, hence the name. Most patients recover within a few months, but there can be complications such as ventricular tachycardia, cardiac arrest, and further major adverse cardiac events, and there is a 5 per cent risk of recurrence. Treatment is similar to heart failure management including things like beta blockers, statins, blood thinners and medications used to manage blood pressure.[33]

Another possible reason that women fare worse is that, despite the belief that we are hysterically racing to the doctors endlessly complaining about our health, it seems we don't take our heart risk factors seriously and are therefore in poorer health when we are diagnosed with a heart condition.

This is something that BMS-accredited menopause specialist, Dr Carys Sonnenberg, is on a mission to change. She has been educating fellow doctors on this because it's just so important. Around menopause, she says, we gain weight around the middle and we have those blood profile changes we mentioned before – higher triglycerides and more of the 'bad' LDL cholesterol. Our lean muscle mass starts to decrease, our blood pressure rises – and this is what really gets her riled.

'At the age of 60, about 50% of people women are hypertensive. One of the biggest bugbears I have is discovering someone in my menopause clinic has been seen in general practice and been told they have high blood pressure, and then two or three years later discovering they have not had their blood pressure reading repeated, or received any treatment to reduce their blood pressure.' She says this is something we really need to take ownership of ourselves. 'I advise my patients, "this is your blood pressure. I am now handing responsibility for your blood pressure to you. I would like you to know what it should be, when you should next have it checked, and what numbers you're looking at." In that way the patient is involved in what is important to protect their future health.'

She believes this empowers them to advocate for themselves, and unfortunately if my experience is anything to go by, you must be able to do this – it's a necessity. While one side of my family is struck down by early onset Alzheimer's, the other side drops dead like flies from strokes. My grandfather had one and died, my uncle had one and died, and my father had one and was incapacitated on the left side of his body and never fully recovered his speech or movement. He had high blood pressure. I have high blood pressure. I don't smoke, I do exercise (although I am a little overweight), I am on MHT and I have an excellent diet. I monitor it and even though I was on a tablet for it, it started to progressively go higher and higher. One night I went up to the hospital because I just didn't feel 'right' and it was up to 165/98. When I got there, I was a little dizzy and they took me through. This was during COVID and while I was waiting alone in the corridor I had a panic attack, burst into tears and I could feel myself flushing and turning red, so by the time they came to get me I looked like a beetroot. I have rosacea so when I flush it makes a pattern similar to that of a heavy drinker. When they took my blood pressure, it was up to 185/120 – yet, despite that, the whole time I was there, the conversation centred on how much alcohol I drank. When they discharged me, they gave me a prescription for thiamine – a B group vitamin that they give to alcoholics. I received no advice on my blood pressure.

For nearly two years after that I literally fought with my doctor to get them to change the dose and type of medications I was taking. My blood pressure was regularly higher than 150/90 but they told me that anything 'around' 140/90 was OK and mine wasn't 'too high'. I'd tell them there were new guidelines out that set lower limits and, given my family history, I'd like mine to be closer to the norm of 120/80 – or at least under 130/90. It took two years for me to convince them to up my medication, and eventually another was added. But Dr Sonnenberg is right – know your numbers and what's recommended as normal, because you may have to advocate for yourself.

Many of us understand the importance of a healthy diet and regular exercise to try to maintain a healthy weight, but there is a lot more to consider than what the scales say, she says. We need to look at where we store our body fat, as this influences our health risk. We know women tend to gain around 10 kg around menopause and tend to store it more often than not around the waist, stored as subcutaneous fat and visceral fat. This 'central obesity' is linked with tissue inflammation, which results in oxidative stress and leads to insulin resistance. Post menopausal women tend to store fat in locations such as the liver and muscle. So their body composition changes. And, we may lose lean mass (everything other than fat, such as muscles, bone and other tissues).

Interestingly, simply measuring body weight and working out a body mass index (BMI) does not show that these changes in body composition are happening. This is because measuring a BMI is not a direct measure of central obesity. NICE guidelines suggest adults with a BMI under 35 kg/m^2 use a waist-to-height ratio, as well as their BMI, to help estimate central adiposity. Both measurements can then be used to predict health risks. If your BMI is less than 35, a healthy central adiposity is a waist-to-height ratio of 0.4–0.49 (indicating no increased health risk). A waist-to-height ratio of 0.5 or greater indicates an increased risk of developing type 2 diabetes and cardiovascular disease.

And we're already seeing the results of our increasing girths. The number of women with pre-diabetes tripled between 2013 and 2018.[34] In the US in 2021 there were around 96 million people with prediabetes and 38.1 million adults with type 2 diabetes. Men were slightly ahead of women with 19.8 per cent of men being diagnosed as opposed to 18.3 per cent of women, but we're catching up fast.[35] Globally cardiovascular disease is the leading cause of death and accounts for almost 50 per cent of all deaths in women worldwide, Dr Sonnenberg says.

So to summarise the metabolic changes during the menopause transition, we have:

- weight gain (especially around the middle)
- loss of bone and muscle
- increased subclinical atherosclerosis (plaques in the blood vessels)
- an increase in insulin resistance
- a change in blood lipids that create a 'proatherogenic lipid profile', increasing the risk of plaque building up in the arteries. The total cholesterol, low density lipoprotein (LDL-C) and triglycerides all rise.

So checking your lipids and your blood pressure is important as you might need medications to lower them, Sonnenberg says, as is maintaining a healthy weight and exercising. Exercise has the added benefit of improving the ratio of 'good' to 'bad' cholesterol as well. But what about statins – wont they do that?

Yes, before menopause statins work very well and have been shown to reduce the number of heart attacks and deaths from heart attacks, but the American College of Cardiology has released a study that suggests that after menopause they may not be as effective and blockages in the carotid artery build up quickly. That doesn't mean they don't work, so don't throw your meds in the rubbish bin – it seems there are multiple things simultaneously at work here in the larger and smaller vascular networks – and this is just one study.

They studied 579 women matched with men with the same baseline coronary artery calcium or CAC score (a measure of the amount of plaque build-up in the arteries) as well as other risk factors (age, race, diabetes or high blood pressure status) who were taking statins to control their cholesterol. There were three groups with low, medium and high CAC scores at the start when they were first scanned, and a year later they were scanned again – and the women didn't do well. The women in the first two groups had double the rise in CAC scores in comparison to men, leading the researchers to surmise that dropping oestrogen levels were a possible reason. The women were not on MHT which is known to have a protective effect on the heart but it is not currently recommended as primary prevention for a heart disease.

The researchers wrote: 'After menopause, women have much less estrogen and shift to a more testosterone-heavy profile . . . This affects the way your body stores fat, where it stores fat and the way it processes fat; it even affects the way your blood clots. And all of those increase your risk for developing heart disease.'

Another reason suggested for the rapid increase in this group of women was that the dose of the statins they were on was no longer sufficient for the changes that are associated with menopause on our cardiovascular system. In its 'call to action', the European Atherosclerosis Society called for greater attention to be paid to the treatment of lipids in women.

So, what can you do? A lot, says Dr Sonnenberg – and it's vital that you do.

She says, 'Stopping smoking, a healthy diet and regular physical exercise, with a combination of exercises such as balance, flexibility, stretching, endurance, and progressive strengthening are all super important.'

The final thing to tackle is the triglycerides. Dr Sonnenberg says MHT can help a little with this, but it all comes back to lifestyle.

'Cardiovascular disease in women remains understudied and diagnosed, under-recognised and undertreated. We need so much more research in this area to optimise care for women with heart disease and improve cardiovascular outcomes for women around the world,' Sonnenberg adds.

But you can take steps to improve your risk profile and even if you are on MHT – don't rely on that alone.

You can:

- make sure your diet is as good as it could be – preferably a Mediterranean diet, high in fruit and veggies with lots of fish and lean meats
- exercise regularly
- don't smoke – it affects blood vessels, and
- reduce your stress levels.

9

Did you just say my clitoris might shrink?

Vaginas. Anyone who knows me will know it's one of my favourite topics. We seem to have a lot of 'last taboos' in women's health, and vaginal and vulval health are two of them. But, at last, these are getting some attention. I'd like to think I've played a small hand in this. Much to my family's embarrassment, I've spent a good number of years talking publicly about them and their pelvic floor neighbours, including my own. I claim it as a small victory that my husband now knows the difference between a Volvo and a vulva.

But he's not alone in his ignorance of female anatomy. A 2019 YouGov study found that 'Half of Brits don't know where the vagina is,' according to its headline, and while you may be thinking they were only talking to men, it was women too.[1] To be fair, their headline may be a little misleading because they were actually asked to name the parts of the female genitalia on a diagram, so they may have known where the vagina or other parts were, but not what the correct name was. YouGov was, however, quite generous in the answers it accepted from the 2010 respondents, allowing for example 'wee hole' for urethra and 'lips' for the 'labia'. But even with this generosity it found that only 55 per cent of women and 41 per cent of men could even vaguely name the vagina and only 45 per cent of women and 39 per cent of men knew what the urethra was called. The labia fared slightly better with 57 per cent of women and 48 per cent of men able to name them. Fortunately, for sexual pleasure purposes, 71 per cent of women and 69 per cent of men could name the clitoris. (Whether they can find it in practice is, of course, another matter, but it is important given only around 15–25 per cent of women climax from penetrative sex alone, depending on whose study you're looking at.)

Does it matter if people can't name their 'bits'? Yes. One of the reasons why I've spent so many years talking about vaginas and vulvas is because if we can't name the parts that we're having problems with, we're sending our doctors on a fishing expedition to find out where the problem is. Turning up and saying I have pain in my 'vajajay', 'foo', 'poontang', 'batcave', 'penis fly trap', 'notorious V.A.G' or even 'frothy creek' (you can thank Buzzfeed for that one[2]) doesn't really give them a precise place to start their investigation. All these terms indicate the problem is internal (in the vagina), but if it's on the outside you've literally led them on a dead-end expedition down your 'love tunnel', and wasted precious time. And with the average consultation being only ten minutes long, you don't have time to waste!

Unfortunately, the media appears to be equally as ignorant. When *Sex Education* star Gillian Anderson trod lightly down the red carpet at the Golden Globes in January 2024 wearing a dress embroidered with vulva motifs, very few of the media organisations that covered the event got it right. Headlines screamed 'vagina dress'. Even *Women & Home*, whose name suggests its target audience is women, only got it half right.[3] They seemed to think the terms 'vagina' and 'vulva' were interchangeable. They wrote:

> The vulva pattern on Gillian Anderson's Golden Globes dress took a mind-boggling 150 hours to embroider.
>
> That's over 40 vaginas, at roughly 3.5 hours each.

Maybe they were having a bet each way.

GP and women's health advocate Dr Aziza Sesay is a huge fan of calling a vulva a vulva and is known across the UK for her black and brown crocheted props that represent people of diverse ethnic backgrounds who often feel unrepresented. They also show that labia come in all different shapes and sizes so people understand that they don't have to 'look' a certain way – we're all unique.

She says there are a few reasons why it's important that we know and use correct names. 'The first is so we remove the taboo and more women will come forward about their genital health and any symptoms they may have, because there are so many people who are suffering in silence because of the shame and stigma. The second is so they can appropriately name the area where they are having symptoms, and so we can educate our children and empower them to have good relationships with their own body and come forward about any issues they have and don't end up suffering in silence, too. The third reason is for their protection from sexual predators, because we know they are less likely to target children who know the correct words because they've probably been educated about abuse.'

But it's not just names that we're confused with. The YouGov survey also found we have some significant hygiene issues and don't really understand that the vagina can pretty well take care of itself. In fact, it is often referred to as a 'self-cleaning unit'. Much like your gut or skin, your vagina has its own microbiota, with a mixture of both good and bad bacteria that generally live happily together and keep it functioning well. These bacteria (along with adequate oestrogen) help maintain a slightly acidic pH environment – about 3.8–4.5 on the pH scale, where 1 is melt your face off/dissolve your food, 7 is neutral like water and 14 is a very strong alkaline – think drain cleaner. This slightly acidic pH helps protect the vagina from invading and unwanted bacteria.

That's not the only trick up its sleeve. The vagina, cervix and the Bartholin glands all produce mucus. This is usually thin, clear or off-whitish, with perhaps a mild odour. It flushes out the dead skin cells as well as semen from the vagina, keeping it 'clean' – I put that in inverted commas because I don't think the vagina should be called 'clean' as it plays into the narrative that it requires attention and without it, it's 'dirty'. To me these terms are at best marketing tools and at worst derisory, harking back to the historical views of women in society that have defined us for centuries and perpetuate feelings of shame when it comes to menstruation or vaginal fluids. 'Healthy' might be a better option, but clearly the 'clean' message resonates as almost half (46 per cent) of the 997 respondents who answered this section of the survey said they thought the vagina needed to be washed with soap, and 14% of them thought it should be washed with soap every single day.

By age group, there wasn't a huge difference but the 55+ group seemed to be the most 'pro' washing at 16 per cent. Thankfully it seems that not all their kids are listening to them as only 10 per cent of 18–24-year-olds and 14 per cent of 25–34-year-olds thought it was a necessity. This, however, provides fertile ground for those who are selling intimate hygiene products. If they can convince the other 54 per cent of women they need soapy, rose-scented products inside and out, they've doubled their already lucrative market. How lucrative? According to Future Finance Inc. the global women's intimate care market in 2024 was worth $30.21 billion and it's expected to grow to $44.36 billion over the next decade[4] (see Chapter 6).

But washing your vagina doesn't come without a cost. Sometimes known as 'douching', it can set off a chain of unsavoury changes that disrupt the very mechanisms – that microbiota and the pH – that the vagina has built to keep you infection free and comfortable.

One of my go-to doctors on all things vaginal during peri- and postmenopause is Dr Juliet Balfour, a GP and British Menopause Society-accredited menopause specialist and trainer. She is also a member of its medical advisory council as well as my menopause charity, the Menopause Research and Education Fund's medical advisory board.

Her advice? Throw your soap in the bin – it has no place inside of your vagina or outside. 'Soap can be very drying so wash external areas with a non-soap cleanser, emollient or warm water alone. Don't wash more than once or twice daily. If the vulva feels dry or itchy, a suitable emollient like Hydromol can be applied after washing as well. Some women benefit from a suitable vaginal moisturiser and a suitable lubricant is recommended for sex.' (More on lubes and moisturisers later.)

But it's not just washing that has an effect, declining oestrogen also plays a significant role. 'The lack of oestrogen in the vagina leads to many changes such as reduced blood flow, reduced lubrication, less elasticity and a thinning of the mucosa.' Dr Balfour explains, 'The changed vaginal cells that are now shed contain less glycogen which lactobacilli in the vagina need to produce lactic acid. With less glycogen available, the pH rises, leading to a change in the vaginal microbiome including more pathogenic bacteria such as E. coli that can increase the risk of urinary tract infections.' That's quite a set of things for one small canal to deal with! Lack of oestrogen in the vulva also leads to reduced blood flow, reduced sensation and thinning of the tissues, leading to soreness and even splitting of the skin, plus the labia and clitoris can shrink. (You said what – the clitoris shrinks? More on that little bombshell later too.)

I mentioned 'comfortable' earlier. Anything that disrupts the balance could result not just in infections but a constant itching and/or burning of the skin, and that's not fun. Take it from me, I know, and this is why I spend a lot of time talking about vaginas and vulvas.

Let me take you back to the early 1980s. I studied anatomy at university and was even a tutor for first year med students in my final year. I only remember having one lecture on female genitalia and the reproductive system in general, and it was very useful. I remember the lecturer standing up, turning sideways, bending forward about 45 degrees and leaning his legs backward slightly, stretching his arms out behind him wiggling his fingers. He said his legs were the vagina, his trunk was the uterus, his arms were the fallopian tubes and his fingers were the fimbriae, the little finger-like tentacles at the end of the fallopian tubes that help usher an ovum, or egg, from the ovary into the tube to carry it to the uterus in the hope that it could be fertilised and make a baby. His physical demonstration was to show that, unlike the diagrams we often see of the female reproductive system, the vagina and uterus aren't standing up straight like a cross, instead the vagina tilts slightly backwards while the uterus generally leans forwards (unless retroverted) with the bladder underneath it, parts of the intestines and colon are above it and the rectum runs down behind it. The ovaries are towards the spine and that's why the fallopian tubes are heading backwards in that direction.

In the practical sessions in the anatomy lab, we spent a lot of time dissecting various human limbs and organs and I give a huge thank you to all those who donate their bodies to science. We chopped up a lot of penises and scrotums and they were fascinating, but I don't recall ever dissecting or even closely examining a single section of the female reproductive tract – not a single vagina, uterus or ovary. We looked at where these organs sat in the pelvis but we never actually handled them. And, I don't recall ever even looking at the external genitalia of a corpse, and that's probably a vision that would have stuck in my mind!

Let's not forget that, while the clitoris has been discussed since ancient times, it was apparently 'discovered' or at least first described in the mid-1500s by Italian anatomist Realdo Colombo. I say apparently, there is argument over who 'discovered' it first. That said, you'd think there'd be quite a lot of interest in such a wonderful little organ whose sole purpose it seems, is to give pleasure, but it then took about another 455 years or so for its full extent to be revealed by Australian urologist, Helen O'Connell, in 2005. (What does that say about misogyny in medicine?) So, suffice to say, when I went through anatomy it was just a bundle of nerves under a little hood that we never actually looked at, not the extensive organ that we know and love, that swells with blood like a penis running along the base of the pelvic floor.

We did study the changes to the sexual organs at puberty and during pregnancy and the hormones involved, but we didn't study the changes at menopause beyond being told periods ended. That was that. No more to say.

I never gave any of this much thought until I hit menopause some 30 years later and discovered what it was like to be 'uncomfortable'. What no one had told me – and I still can't quite believe this having spent some 20 years in medical publishing after leaving the Australian Broadcasting Corporation – not a single soul told me my vagina was going to dry up, the skin on my labia would itch, burn and tear, and my clitoris could shrink![5] No one said a word. As you can imagine, that revelation was quite a shock – especially the last bit.

And, contrary to what an industry that's designed to 'tighten' your vagina will tell you, your vagina is not 'lax' and resembling something like a wind tunnel that you could land a jet in and test its engines, with labial tissue flapping around like a set of old theatre curtains at the entrance. The vagina shrinks in length. Its blood supply reduces, its walls become thinner and the folds, or rugae, that play a role in the maintenance of a healthy microbiota and give the vagina the elasticity it needs to stretch for childbirth or sex, disappear. Some women may say they get less pleasure from sex as the sensation has decreased and for others sex may become painful. And it can be a slow, insidious set of creeping changes that you can easily brush off as something else – which is exactly what I did. So, I'll tell you my story to save you from making the same mistake. (By the way, let me just add two things here: first, some women say they have the best sex of their lives after menopause, so it's not all doom and gloom; and second, if your male partner tells you your vagina is no longer the nice snug fit it used to be it may be worth reminding him that penises shrink too, so in this case, 'it may not be me, darling, it could be you!')

During perimenopause I had 'a little bit of dryness' sometimes, but nothing to write home about. I went through menopause at about 50 (I don't actually remember when exactly my last period was) and slowly, over the next two to three years, I started to notice that my labia were increasingly itchy and burning. It felt a bit like the beginnings of thrush, which I'd been prone to in earlier years, but it never quite developed into a full-blown bout. Each time I headed to the nearest pharmacy to grab yet another tube of the antifungal, clotrimazole. I was living on the stuff and it did provide a bit of relief for a short period of time, but that burn and itch just kept coming back. After buying what was probably my fourth tube in six months the pharmacist said to me 'you really should get that checked' but being a bit of a smarty-pants, I replied 'I think I know my own body' – only to find that I actually didn't. I had no idea.

Things continued to get worse to the point that about four years in, my labia were so sore that it was painful to sit, walk or exercise. I couldn't wear jeans anymore, and finding suitable underwear became a significant problem. Unless it was super soft cotton it was a no go. Countless types were bought, with most making their way to the back of the drawer very quickly, never to see the light of day again. The burning and itching would wake me at night and if I was walking I would constantly have to find a quiet spot to stop and literally re-adjust myself so I could walk on. Sex, well, you can pretty much forget about that – even though dryness wasn't my biggest issue, the labia formed a formidable and off-putting barrier. Think: 'penis wrapped in sandpaper', and you'll know where I'm coming from. So, when I hear people saying 'it's just a bit of dryness' – I beg to differ. (If you're a man and you're reading this – reverse that image and think vagina lined with sandpaper, and not the fine grained stuff, and you'll get the picture.)

But it's not just physical discomfort, there's also a psychological aspect. I found menopause confronting enough with the low mood, mood swings, anxiety, loss of confidence, brain fog, weight gain, hair loss and everything from my jowls to my belly heading south. Add to that the myriad of questions about our role in society once you can no longer reproduce (since that's what we seem to be valued for), and I was tearing myself apart, and I remember sitting on my bed in tears thinking; 'God, it's come to this, I can't walk, I can't sit, I can't even have sex anymore, what can I do?' I know this may sound over-the-top or mildly 'hysterical' (you know how we love that word) to some, it but made me question the purpose of existence post-reproduction, particularly my own. I'm not saying it was an existential crisis, but I had to re-evaluate and recalibrate, and I now wonder if this is what people who've found menopause to be a liberating experience have managed well (see Chapter 12 for more on the 'good' menopause).

When you put all of these symptoms we attribute to menopause together, it can shake you to the core and make you question your sense of self. I'll admit there may have been elements of vanity in this for me, but it's so much more. It's your inner self-confidence. I'm not talking about your ability to public speak or take part in office discussions or even function at work, but something much deeper. I felt isolated, alone – it was very much like grief, that pit in the stomach emptiness you feel when you've lost someone you care about, in this case, yourself. Why? Because society values youth and tells us that a woman's basic purpose is to reproduce. But what happens when you no longer can?

My own vagina and its dryness, itching and burning had affected my relationship. It took me two years to work up enough courage to tell my partner 'it wasn't him, it was me', because I was embarrassed. For many couples, various myths can come to the fore here. Women may think that if a man's penis isn't 'hard', he's no longer interested in her, when the reason could actually be a tell-tale sign of erectile dysfunction. Men may think that if a woman isn't 'wet' then she's no longer interested in him, when it could be exactly what I've just described – hormones playing havoc with your genitalia. Fortunately, my partner was hugely understanding and I thank him for it, but not everyone's is.

Over the past seven years or so that I've been talking about vaginal health and menopause I've had some tear-jerking messages from women who had found themselves in a similar situation but didn't have the same support – in fact, quite the opposite. One in particular that sticks in my mind is a woman who was asking what she should do because her husband didn't believe her when she said that sex was painful, and he was threatening to divorce her if she didn't oblige. This is why this discussion is so important – no one should be in that position.

But unfortunately, they are. I ran a poll in 2023 on sexual health in postmenopause for those aged 55+ and analysed the first 200 responses. I'm not in any way holding this up as a piece of science but rather as a snap shot shedding light on the extent of the problem. Of those aged 55–64 (the vast majority of respondents) who said they were postmenopausal:

- 68 per cent said they had low libido (a loss of interest in sex)
- 56 per cent said they had vaginal dryness
- 45 per cent said they had itching and burning
- 25 per cent said sex was painful
- 13 per cent had recurrent UTIs
- 11 per cent had tearing or bleeding after sex.

One-third hadn't had sex for more than a year with 58 per cent of them saying it was because sex was too painful. Of the third who had had sex in the past seven days 86.7 per cent said it was painful. Let me just say that again, 86.7 per cent of women who had had sex in the past week were enduring pain. It really puts a whole new perspective on the phrase 'lie back and think of England'. But it doesn't have to be this way – the right advice and treatments can make a huge difference.

These vaginal changes are part of what's known as the Genitourinary Syndrome of Menopause (GSM). It's not a term that rolls off the tongue but it's marginally better than its predecessor, 'vaginal atrophy'. Why the change of nomenclature? Because it doesn't just affect the vagina, that drop in oestrogen also affects the vulva, the clitoris, the bladder, urethra (the tube that carries urine from the bladder out of your body) and all the tissues in the pelvic floor as they too have oestrogen receptors and experience reduced blood supply.

The result – it's quite a list I'm afraid:

- Vaginal dryness, itching, soreness and painful sex
- Vulval dryness, itching, soreness, splitting of the skin, reduced sensation, reduced ability to orgasm and painful sex
- An increase in urinary tract infections (UTIs)
- Bladder leakage (stress urinary incontinence)
- Increased frequency – the number of times you have to go, which can be very annoying, especially if you're getting up numerous times a night

- Urge incontinency – the need to go NOW, rushing to the loo and sometimes not making it
- Prolapses.

For these bladder and prolapse issues, pelvic floor physios can be a life-saver. They can work with you on ways to 'retrain' your bladder, strengthen the muscles if that's what you need to help improve a prolapse or prevent it, and they can teach you how to relax the pelvic floor muscles too – as that may be a contributing factor to painful sex. If you can't get to see one on the NHS and you have these issues, saving up for an appointment or two could change your life and it will pay for itself over time – think of all the absorbent underwear (disposable or otherwise) that you won't have to buy!

Depending on whose study you're looking at, GSM symptoms can affect somewhere between 27–84 per cent of women.[6] It's speculated that this variation is due in part to women being too embarrassed to talk about it, but it really is something that they should discuss, Dr Balfour says. 'We know that GSM is under-reported, underdiagnosed and under-treated. It may start in the perimenopause or not for many years after the last period. Unlike most other menopausal symptoms that go eventually, GSM will only worsen with time if not treated. It is important that women have an examination to confirm the diagnosis and exclude other issues that could be causing symptoms such as lichen sclerosus, irritant dermatitis, psoriasis, lichen planus, thrush or cancerous changes.'

What helps?

Current recommendations say that vaginal oestrogen, sometimes called 'topical' or 'local' oestrogen, is the first-line treatment for vaginal symptoms. Yes, these preparations contain oestrogen in different forms or a testosterone precursor called DHEA, but they are not considered to be MHT. They are used around the labia if needed and there is very little systemic absorption after the initial loading dose. There is a growing consensus that they are safe for most people and that includes breast cancer patients after their cancer treatment is finished.[7] Women who are taking tamoxifen can use the ultra-low-dose estriol products too (see below), but Dr Balfour says women who are taking aromatase inhibitors 'need to have a discussion with their oncologist to consider their options. Unfortunately, this group of women tend to suffer badly from GSM but local oestrogen is currently not the first-line option. It may be considered on an individual basis depending on symptoms and after explaining the uncertainties. More research on the use of local oestrogen or prasterone (DHEA) pessaries is desperately needed to establish the safest treatment for this group of patients.'

When it comes to gynaecological cancers it again has mostly green lights but there are a few where it is recommended with caution or advised against, according to the latest BMS guidelines.[8] The 'with caution' include:

- a type of cancer that can affect the fallopian tubes, ovaries or peritoneal cavity called a low-grade serous stage 2+
- intermediate and high-risk endometrial cancers including oestrogen and progesterone positive and negative cancers once it's become advanced and metastatic cancers.

It's not recommended for uterine sarcoma.

For the vast majority of us though, vaginal oestrogen is safe and effective. Dr Balfour explains that it can be applied via creams or gel (estriol) or vaginal tablets or pessaries (estradiol) that are used initially every day for two to three weeks depending on the preparation, and then a couple of times a week as maintenance after that. If that's not cutting the mustard you can talk to your doctor about using them more often, and yes, the cream or gel can be used on the vulva as well if needed, she says.

There's also a silicone ring that can be inserted into the vagina which gives a constant slow release of estradiol over a three-month period. It can stay in 24/7 and doesn't need to be removed for sex, and it can be used in combination with the estriol cream or gel on the external areas if needed. I have one of these, it's called an Estring in the UK, and it's been a game changer.

There is a daily prasterone (DHEA) pessary which is converted into estradiol and testosterone by the vaginal cells. More research is needed to see when this option is best used.[9]

And there's an oral medication called ospemifene that can help with dryness too. Dr Balfour says this may be a good option for those with dexterity issues who find it difficult to use the pessaries, creams or gels, but it does have some contraindications and a possible side effect of hot flushes.

The most important thing is not to 'do a Fiona' and leave your symptoms for years, but to get on top of it early. Dr Balfour warns, as I have found, 'long-standing changes cannot always be completely reversed' but there can still be improvement.

'The time that takes can vary depending on how long the symptoms have been going on for,' she adds, and it can be a case of trial and error to find what's best for you. 'Some women need to try a few different local oestrogen products until they find one that suits them and that they are happy to use long-term.'

The UK has what I can only describe as an illogical system where medications that are approved for national use then go to local boards across the country to decide if they're suitable for their local population and are the best use of their budget. The result? A postcode lottery where the 'the list of drugs that clinicians can prescribe does vary from area to area in the UK so not all options are available to everyone,' Balfour says. This needs to change. It's cheap and effective and should be available to all who need it.

Balfour says there are many myths about vaginal oestrogen that need to be put to bed.

1. You only need local oestrogen for three months or until your symptoms subside.

'Not true,' she says, 'unfortunately that oestrogen isn't coming back on its own and the symptoms will only get worse over time, so this treatment is for life.'

2. You don't need it if you are taking systemic MHT.

'Again, not true. Many women find that systemic oestrogen doesn't provide enough help for their vaginal symptoms, so they can use both. The amount of oestrogen in vaginal products is tiny, so they won't be overdosing on oestrogen.' Those using local oestrogen alone do not need to take a progestogen for endometrial protection, unlike those on systemic MHT.

3. Vaginal oestrogen carries the same risks as systemic MHT.

If you read the product information leaflets inside the box you will find they list a lot of possible risks including an increased risk of stroke, blood clots and various cancers. Dr Balfour says it is important to point out that this part of the patient information leaflet is inaccurate. 'It lists many risks that simply do not apply to local oestrogen but sadly patients may read this when they get home and then decide not to try it' (see Chapter 11).

4. You only need vaginal oestrogen if you're sexually active.

I've heard women say many times that their doctors told them that since they weren't in a relationship or sexually active they didn't need it – and that's simply not the case. Your relationship status is not relevant.

As Balfour says, 'Many women have vaginal, vulval and urinary symptoms most of the time, unrelated to whether they are sexually active or not.'

Which brings me to the final myth that needs busting here, the 'use it or lose it' argument. It's a theory that is commonly touted, based initially on a 2011 study that found that people who were sexually active reported less vaginal dryness and pain during sex. Those who had pain during sex – dyspareunia – had less sex, but they didn't necessarily complain about dryness, and there are lots of other reasons why there could be pain during sex including overly tight pelvic floor muscles, labial tearing, burning and itching, and trauma, to name a few. The researchers noted that others had hypothesised that being sexually active could be a way of preventing pain during sex developing as it could, in theory, help maintain a well-lubricated vagina – hence 'use it or lose it'. But they concluded more research was needed.[10] What this argument fails to take into account is that people who had less sex weren't avoiding it for fun, but because it was painful, perhaps for any of those reasons above. There is no doubt that sex temporarily improves blood flow to the sexual organs, but there is no evidence to say that it will help maintain lubrication production over time and prevent vaginal dryness which is caused by declining oestrogen levels – and you can't bonk (or bang, depending on where you are) your way out of that. Saying your vaginal dryness and subsequent painful sex is due to you not having had enough sex could effectively be seen as victim blaming. If sex is painful, you are less likely to have sex – simple as that.

Bladder blues

But what about the bladder, can these topical preparations help too?

Dr Rachel Rubin, a US-based board-certified urologist, argues 'yes' – without a doubt. She is the winner of my 2023 headline of the year award for her commentary in Medscape entitled 'Vaginal dryness can be fatal. No, really.'[11] How, you ask? She explains: 'The thing that kills women is recurrent urinary tract infections (UTIs). Did you know that UTIs account for 7 million visits and hospitalizations annually [in the US] and 25% of all infections in older people? In fact, apparently one third of the total Medicare expenditure is around UTIs. Not preventing UTIs is costing our healthcare system an enormous amount of money and resources,' she wrote.

The Agency for Healthcare Research and Quality does indeed report that sepsis costs US hospitals a lot. It says hospital costs for sepsis admissions increased by 66.8% from 2016 to 2021 to a massive $52.1 billion.[12]

And it's not just the US with big bills. In the UK treating sepsis rings up an estimated annual bill of somewhere between £7.6 and £10.2 billion, according to a report done for the Sepsis Trust.[13] It says around 48,000 people die from sepsis in the UK each year and 11 million globally. In England in the 2023–24 financial year there were just under 120,000 admissions to hospital.[14] And a 2004 study says sepsis is responsible for more deaths than prostate cancer, breast cancer and AIDS combined.[15]

These are aggregated figures for all types of sepsis, but one of the most common causes of sepsis is UTIs, and the elderly, particularly women, are most susceptible. One study looked at the number of UTIs women had over the past five years and found that 30 per cent of those over the age of 65 had at least one UTI in the preceding year and 60 per cent had had one in the previous five years.[16] It's estimated that 24 per cent of sepsis cases in older people (over 65 years of age) are due to UTIs, an NHS report claims.[17] Our greater risk for UTI is primarily due to our anatomy. Our urethra is a lot shorter than our male counterparts and it's a lot closer to our anus. Enterobacteriaceae and E. coli are two of the main bugs that cause UTIs. They're regular residents in our intestines where they live quite happily, but they do hitch a ride outside in our poo. Unfortunately, our bladders don't like them quite so much, so when one of them takes up residency there it can wreak havoc. (That's why wiping from front to back after we go to the toilet is so important!) Add in the lack of oestrogen and changes to the microbiome and you've got a perfect storm. 'That lack of oestrogen leads to shrinkage of our labia, reducing their protective effect against infection, plus the walls of the urethra lose their stickiness so the urethra is more open to infection,' Dr Balfour says.

Preventing sepsis is vital, not just because of cost, but because 30 to 40 per cent of those who go on to develop severe sepsis will die,[18] and those who survive can sometimes be left with damage to internal organs and ongoing health issues. That's why vaginal dryness can be fatal.

Here we go again – recurrent UTIs

UTI recurrence is an issue too. You have recurrent UTIs if you have two or more in six months or three in a year. Depending on which study you look at, around 20–30 per cent of younger women will have recurrent UTIs but that figure almost doubles to 55 per cent in women aged over 65. But what may surprise you, or won't, is there are actually very few studies looking at UTI recurrence in postmenopausal women. When I entered 'recurrent UTI postmenopause' or 'postmenopausal' into the National Library of Medicine, a huge database of published medical studies, it returned 122 studies. When I searched the term 'erectile dysfunction' I got back 30,416. So, 100 per cent of women go through menopause, 30 per cent of those will have UTIs, 55 per cent of them will have them a couple of times a year, but just 122 studies have been done on it, even though somewhere between one and four in ten will develop sepsis and 30–40 per cent of them will die. It may be a cheap shot, but around 36 per cent of men aged 44–55 and 50 per cent of men aged over 65 or more will experience erectile dysfunction, none of them will die as a direct result of it.[19]

But it's not just being female, ageing and hygiene that are at play here. Vaginal dryness also has a role. And this brings us back to Dr Rubin's point – giving women topical, vaginal oestrogen could go a long way to reducing the incidence of UTIs in peri- and postmenopausal women.

One study reviewed the medications prescribed to 5,600 women in the US aged between 60 and 80 (median age 70.4) with low oestrogen levels.[20] They were given vaginal oestrogen to prevent recurrent UTIs and the study found the number of infections fell from 3.9 to 1.8 in the year after the topical oestrogen was prescribed – that's a 51.9 per cent reduction in UTIs. Just over 55 per cent of patients had one UTI and 31.4 per cent had none.

That's a significant reduction, achieved through something very cheap and simple, yet it's not one that's very often discussed. In fact, the most recent NICE guidelines on menopause (2024) refers practitioners to its guidance on preventing UTIs where it says: 'Consider vaginal oestrogen for recurrent UTI if behavioural and personal hygiene measures alone are not effective or not appropriate.'[21]

What are those personal hygiene measures? According to the NHS, they are:

- Wipe from front to back when you go to the toilet.
- Keep the genital area clean and dry.
- Drink plenty of fluids, particularly water – so that you pee regularly.
- Wash the skin around the vagina with water before and after sex.
- Pee as soon as possible after sex.
- Promptly change nappies or incontinence pads if they're soiled.

Given there are specific changes around menopause that affect women's risk of developing recurrent UTIs that put them at a higher risk of sepsis and death, and vaginal oestrogen appears to provide a cheap and effective way of reducing the risk, why isn't it a first-line treatment? Why is it only 'considered' when all other hygiene measures have failed? Is there an assumption that around the age of menopause women simply forget basic personal hygiene, wiping back to front and never washing? Is brain fog to blame?

I've had messages from women who have parents in nursing homes asking what they can do in cases where the nursing home has decided to 'stop mum's vaginal oestrogen' because they say 'she doesn't need it any more'. Apart from the fact that she was obviously prescribed it because she did need it, and that lost oestrogen isn't going to magically reappear, it's hard to garner why the nursing home would think she no longer needed it. Studies show that 10 per cent of women over the age of 65 report having had a UTI within the past 12 months, and this rises to almost 30 per cent in women over the age of 85 years,[22] so surely that kind of decision is putting mum at risk.

It would seem to be a short-sighted decision based on local cost without taking into account the cost to the hospital system if mum ends up being admitted, and if she survives, the cost of the antibiotics she's going to have to take over and over again. Not to mention the risk of death. Around 4 per cent will die from it and that rises to 10 per cent for those aged over 95, according to an NHS England report.[23] Why go there when letting her keep her topical oestrogen would be so much easier? And as Dr Balfour says, 'a common cause of new onset or worsening confusion in elderly women is urinary tract infections', and this can put them at risk of falls and broken hips, not to mention further reduce their independence.

'It is safe and indeed essential that women continue to use local (vaginal) oestrogen long term,' she says. 'Age is no barrier to starting it. As GSM can start many years after the menopause, both women and doctors may not attribute the symptoms to lack of oestrogen. My mother had no symptoms at all until the age of 84 when she suddenly developed awful GSM.'

Dr Rubin says vaginal oestrogen has multiple benefits and we just aren't using it as broadly as we should be. 'It prevents UTIs and actually works like sildenafil (Viagra) because it can help orgasm and reduce pain with sex.'

Interestingly vaginal oestrogen may also help with certain types of incontinence with some studies showing vaginal oestrogen may improve the bladder's microbiota, which may help with an overactive bladder.[24] A Cochrane review that looked at 34 trials with 19,676 incontinent women, 1,464 of whom were given topical oestrogen, found that 'significantly more women who received local (vaginal) oestrogen for incontinence reported that their symptoms improved compared to placebo'.[25]

In the UK, you can now buy a vaginal cream or pessary over the counter from a pharmacy, but there are limitations on who can buy it. You have to be postmenopausal and over the age of 50. And even though it is considered to be safe for people who have had breast cancer, you have to have no history of that to buy it at a chemist. Putting an age limit also means anyone who has gone through premature or early menopause can't buy it. There's also a cost factor here. It's not cheap at around £29/month for the pessaries and £20/month for a small tube of estriol cream, so there are equity issues too. People on low incomes may find this prohibitive.

You can get it on the NHS but the amount of it prescribed (or the number of items prescribed) are much lower than those for systemic MHT, which is interesting as it's said only 30 per cent or so of women will have severe vasomotor menopause symptoms, one of the main reasons why it's prescribed, but up to 84 per cent will have vaginal symptoms. From October 2023 to September 2024 open prescribing data shows the Estring was dispensed 9,255 times at a cost of £289,466 and Vagirux was issued 371,557 times with a cost to the NHS of £4,281,406. Sandrena and Oestrogel, two systemic oestrogen products, were dispensed 234,870 and 988,329 times at a cost of £3,439,141 and £14,025,716 respectively. In other words, when it comes to these two products, around four times more systemic items were prescribed than topical ones.

Other things that can help include vaginal moisturisers and lubricants. Finding a good one though is no easy task, especially in a market that's unregulated. Yes, you would think that anything that goes in or near your vagina would be closely scrutinised for efficacy and safety, but sadly, you'd be very, very wrong again. If you're not making any major claims about prevention or cure, it slips (no pun intended) somewhere between cosmetic products and toiletries.

The man who has done a huge amount of research in this area is Nick Panay, an honorary professor and consultant gynaecologist in London who is regarded as one of the leading authorities on menopause. He and his colleagues have conducted extensive research into the products that are on the market, looking at what's in them, their pH (acid balance) and their osmolality – a measure of the concentration of dissolved particles in a fluid, or its concentration.

Basically, if the concentration of some ingredients is too high it can damage sensitive tissues.

According to the WHO,[26] the osmolality of a personal lubricant, a product that gives temporary relief and/or makes sex possible when dryness is an issue, should not exceed 380 mOsm/kg or it could damage the delicate lining of the vagina. Unfortunately, very few preparations meet that level and because of that, Professor Panay explains in the study, 'an upper limit of 1,200 mOsm/kg is generally deemed acceptable in practice'. But the tests he and his colleagues ran on 32 products showed that just 12 came in under 1,200 and only eight of those were under 380 mOsm/kg.[27]

As we've said, when it comes to the vagina the normal pH range is 3.8–4.5 and for the rectum it's around 7.0. Again, very few products made the grade, some coming at levels that animal data suggests is 'unacceptable' for human use. That would be anything with a pH of 3 or below. That's a strong acid like lemon juice or vinegar – fine in a salad dressing but probably not your first choice for a vaginal product. His test showed that just 10 of the 32 products for vaginal or rectal use were within the right pH range with two under a pH of 3 and one at 3.5.

When it comes to the ingredients themselves, you'd think, what could possibly go wrong? Well, quite a lot it seems.

Some products contain parabens which don't have a great reputation for putting on your skin these days, let alone inside your vagina, due to their possible links with endocrine disruption and cancer.

Glycols – glycerol, glycerine and propylene glycol – are products that are commonly used in the cosmetic industry because they improve hydration when applied to the skin. But it's not quite the same inside the vagina. Professor Panay explains that if glycols are in too high a concentration they can irritate the vaginal mucosa or lining. They've been shown in animal studies to increase susceptibility to the herpes simplex 2 virus (HSV2) and a combination of 'propylene glycol, glycerine and methylparaben has also been shown to kill Lactobacillus crispatus in vitro, which is the dominant bacterial species in the vaginal microbiome that helps maintain a healthy mucosal barrier and acidic pH,' the study says. These products have been associated with outbreaks of bacterial vaginosis and thrush.

Sam Evans knows this market only too well. She is a former nurse turned sex writer and co-founder of the sex toy company Jo Divine. Her ethos is firmly based on finding and recommending products that are safe for intimate skin, but she says the market is awash with products making all kinds of claims and filled with all kinds of ingredients, many of which have no clinical data backing them for safety on vaginal tissue.

'Be an ingredients detective,' she says. 'If you care about what you eat, use on your face, body and hair, think about what you use intimately. Just because a product is slippery doesn't mean it is suitable for intimate use. I have to say it's not just glycols, glycerin and parabens, we have dyes, perfume, alcohol, glitter and now CBD lubes. All the CBD brands want me to sell them but none has been able to provide any clinical evidence-based research about their impact upon the microbiome of the vagina, plus many of the base carrier ingredients are irritants.'

She's not a great fan of raiding the kitchen cupboard for coconut or olive oil, or some of the oils that are being sold for relieving GSM symptoms, asking how can they do so if they are only recommended for external use? And, she says, remember: oil and latex don't mix. If you're using oil-based products and latex condoms, you're decreasing their effectiveness.

All in all, it's a minefield out there!

10

Sleep, skin and other things

We spend about one-third of our lives asleep – although around men-opause those hours of blissful rest may seem more like a dream than a reality. Poor sleep is one of the most common complaints women mention, affecting around 50 per cent but that rises to 64 per cent of those who also report having hot flushes.[1] The thing about these hot flushes is that even if they don't wake you up, they can still disrupt your sleep without you knowing.[2] As we saw before, Dr Maki had no idea she was having hot flushes in her sleep until she wore a monitor that detects them.

It's said we should have six to eight hours of sleep, but not get-ting enough can interfere with the way the brain functions, which could see you having difficulty in making decisions or solving prob-lems, controlling your emotions or coping with change. It's also been linked to depression, suicide and risk-taking behaviour, Johns Hopkins Hospital in the US says.[3]

Why is sleep so important?

We might think our brains are having a good rest while we sleep, but they're actually doing a lot of things, including engaging in some serious self-cleaning. It's like a detox dump where all the waste prod-ucts are swept away in a process called glymphatic drainage. This is quite new stuff and it's super interesting. As we know, we have blood coursing through our brains, but it actually only makes up about 10 per cent of the fluid that goes through it. The other fluids are intra-cellular fluid, interstitial fluid and the cerebrospinal fluid, and while we sleep these flood the brain and remove waste products including the beta amyloid and tau proteins that are associated with Alzheimer's disease. They pick these up and flush them out via the lymphatic drainage system.[4] Clever. Research is now underway to look at ways of enhancing the process to reduce the risk of dementia, and Alzheimer's in particular.

So, that's one interesting thing about sleep, but there are others. While we sleep we cycle through various phases that are important for memory consolidation and how refreshed we feel in the morning. These are rapid eye movement (REM) sleep and non-REM sleep, and non-REM sleep has sub-phases.

REM sleep starts about 90 minutes after falling asleep. If you're watching someone during this phase of sleep you might see their eyeballs moving rapidly under the eyelids, and recordings of the brain waves during that time show this stage of sleep is closer to what you'd expect to see if you were awake. During this phase your breathing gets faster and it might be irregular, and your heart rate and blood pressure go up, too. This is when you do most of your dreaming, fortunately though your legs and arms are 'deactivated' for want of a better word, so you usually don't start acting your dreams out. (That said, Mum told me once Dad tried to strangle her in his sleep – but perhaps that's because of her snoring – who knows?) It's thought some memory consolidation takes place during REM sleep but it can also take place in non-REM sleep too. As you age, the amount of time you spend in REM sleep starts to decrease.

When it comes to non-REM sleep there are three phases.

- Stage 1 – this is the changeover from wakefulness to sleep. It's a short period of relatively light sleep when things start to calm – your heartbeat, breathing, eye movements and brain waves start to slow, and your muscles start to relax. It doesn't last long – several minutes or so.
- Stage 2 – this is the light sleep that precedes deep sleep. Everything slows even more, your temperature drops and your eye movements stop. Brainwave activity slows but there are occasional brief bursts of electrical activity. This phase of sleep occurs more than any of the others during the night.
- Stage 3 – this is the deep sleep you need to bounce out of bed and feel refreshed in the morning. It occurs mostly in the first half of the night. You're super relaxed, breathing slowly and it can be hard to wake you up.

Obviously, anything that breaks these phases of sleep is going to impact how well you sleep and how good you feel in the morning. You don't need to be a brain surgeon to work out that drinking a lot of alcohol will interfere with your quality of sleep as your body is trying to get rid of that as well as all the other waste, so it's going to play havoc with this first phase of deep sleep. But other things do too, like having to get up and pee multiple times a night, and those vasomotor symptoms.

A perfect storm – sleep apnoea, vasomotor symptoms and heart health?

You could be forgiven for thinking that those hot flashes and night sweats are an annoyance, but they can do so much more than soak your sheets and ruin your sleep. Not only can they affect your brain health they can also affect your heart, and Dr Maki says they should not be ignored. Studies show they're associated with all the things we've just been talking about in the chapter on bone and heart health – high blood pressure, insulin resistance and bad cholesterol and triglyceride profiles, diabetes, and metabolic syndrome. And, they've been related to changes to the lining of the blood vessels and endothelial dysfunction and early stage of plaque build-up.[5] The exact mechanism isn't yet known – more research is needed but those working in the area believe they could indicate who is at greater risk and in need of targeted interventions to reduce the risk of cardiovascular disease (see Chapter 8).

You may remember that we mentioned in the chapter on brains a condition called sleep apnoea – this is something we usually associate with overweight middle-aged men, but it affects women too, especially after menopause, and its super important that we deal with it. Why? Because not only can it affect your brain health and increase your risk of dementia, it can affect your heart health too and increase your risk of a stroke. And even though it's estimated that somewhere between 47–67 per cent of us will have it,[6] it's massively underdiagnosed in midlife women. So, it's not just overweight middle-aged men – it's us too!

What is sleep apnoea and how do I know if I have it?

It's a condition that interferes with breathing when you sleep. The symptoms include:

- temporarily stopping and restarting breathing
- making gasping, loud snorting or choking/gurgling type noises
- waking up a lot (although, as with the vasomotor symptoms, you may not actually wake up but your sleep is still disturbed)
- snoring loudly.

When you wake up or during the day you may:

- feel tired and yawn a lot
- have difficulty concentrating
- be moody
- have a headache.

You may need to go to a sleep clinic to get it diagnosed, but sometimes the tests can be done at home. They monitor your heart rate, oxygen flow and breathing patterns.

The risk factors for sleep apnoea include:

- being overweight
- not exercising/a sedentary lifestyle
- smoking
- drinking too much.

The take-home here is: if your partner tells you you're snoring, don't take it as an insult. Instead take it as a life-saving health tip and speak to your doctor about what could help. If you live alone, or your partner sleeps like a log, there are apps that can be used to monitor your sleep, but bear in mind these are not approved diagnostic tools. They may give you an indication though, as well as a starting point for your conversation with your doctor.

What are the treatments?

Most people associate sleep apnoea with having to be attached to a CPAP machine that helps you breathe by constantly pumping pressurised air into you, which helps keep your airways open. But there are a number of things you can do to help yourself before reaching that stage and chief among them are losing weight, exercising, cutting down on alcohol and not smoking. (No surprises there.)

Sleeping on your side might help. Some people put a tennis ball in the back of their PJs to stop them from rolling on to their back. Sounds extreme but might be worth a try. There are also wedge-like pillows that can stop you from rolling over, which might be preferable – if the snoring doesn't wake you, a tennis ball in the back probably will!

If you have nasal allergies an antihistamine might help. In some cases, surgery to remove enlarged tonsils can make a difference.[7] There is also an oral device, sort of like a retainer, that helps keep airways open too.[8]

Don't be afraid to talk to your doctor about sleep apnoea for fear of having to spend your nights attached to a less-than-sexy machine – you have options. And it's not just important for your heart and brain health, being sleepy during the daytime means you are at increased risk of an accident when you're driving, or if your job involves operating machinery. You could injure yourself or someone else, so it's really important that you take snoring seriously.

Sleep hygiene

But what about simply getting to sleep and staying that way? We hear a lot about sleep hygiene and having good sleep habits to help improve sleep – many of these you may be familiar with, but just in case you aren't, here they are:

- Set a regular bedtime.
- Reduce screen time if you can, at least a couple of hours before bed.
- Reduce alcohol – you may think it helps you get to sleep but it ruins your sleep quality (let alone contributing to sleep apnoea!).
- Reduce stress.
- Try to get your room nice and dark, and not too hot.
- Don't work in bed or watch TV in bed – experts say bed should be for two things only – sex and sleep. If you do other things there you're telling your brain it's for lots of things apart from sleep and it won't associate bed with sleep as well.
- Get plenty of exercise (although some say leave at least 90 minutes before going to bed).

- Get some morning light if you can.
- Try not to nap in the day as it decreases what's known as the 'sleep drive' – it gets stronger every hour you are awake and helps you to sleep longer and more deeply.
- Cut back on caffeine if that keeps you awake.
- Avoid huge meals before sleep.
- Don't smoke – it's a stimulant.
- Eat a well-balanced diet.

Tips for a good night's sleep

Some people find the following helpful:

- noise-cancelling headphones or white noise apps
- mindfulness and relaxation techniques
- a warm bath
- magnesium supplements in the evening (I'm not advocating any supplements, but some people say they find them useful)
- if you have been prescribed oral progesterone, take it at night as it can make some people drowsy and help with getting to sleep.

Sleep experts say if you can't get back to sleep, instead of lying awake at night, fretting and starting at the ceiling, get up, go somewhere quiet and read or knit or listen to music until you feel the urge to sleep again and then go back to bed. Try to avoid picking up your phone or laptop or watching TV.

What if it's insomnia?

Getting a bad night's sleep every so often is one thing – but then there's insomnia. According to the National Sleep Foundation, insomnia symptoms vary from person to person and some of the common signs are:[9]

- waking up repeatedly or for long periods during the night
- waking up most nights like this
- a short duration of sleep, i.e. waking up too early and not being able to get back to sleep
- waking up feeling as though you haven't slept

- moodiness, irritability, or depression
- cognitive impairment/difficulty concentrating
- relationship problems
- forgetfulness
- increased errors or accidents
- ongoing anxiety about sleep.

If you have insomnia there is a specific type of cognitive behavioural therapy (CBT) that has good evidence behind it for helping people deal with those hours spent away tossing and turning. It's called CBTi and it is available on apps like Sleepio. It is recommended by the NHS and is a course that helps you reframe negative thoughts about being awake at 3 am. For example, if you're thinking 'I'll never function tomorrow', 'I'll lose my job', your stress levels are going to rise and it will be more difficult to get back to sleep. If it's thoughts about life in general that are keeping you awake – constantly problem solving or trouble shooting – it can help you move those aside too. Similarly, if you find it hard to get to sleep and spend time worrying that you never will doze off, it teaches you ways to reframe those thoughts.[10] It also offers tips on retraining your body to increase the hours that you are sleeping so instead of getting 3–4 hours you can slowly extend it over time. The National Sleep Foundation has some good information on this too.[11]

And here's a novel tip – eat kiwi fruit. Apparently, they can help you get to sleep faster and they can add 20 minutes to the length of time you sleep, which may not sound like much but it's better than nothing.[12] To be fair this was a tiny study, but they're good for you anyway, especially for constipation!

Some people find their sleep improves on MHT, and, as mentioned before, if you have oral progesterone, taking it at night can help. Progesterone increases levels of a type of neurotransmitter called GABA which helps keep people calm, so as levels fall around menopause sleep can be affected, which is why taking the progesterone at night helps some people. (Unfortunately, using it vaginally won't deliver this benefit.)

Finally, as Dr Maki says, don't leave those vasomotor symptoms untreated. And, of course, get any bladder issues sorted. That way, at least, there are two less things to disturb you. And, as I've said, pelvic floor physios can work wonders with leakage (stress urinary incontinence) and urgency – that need to go 'NOW!'

Your skin – it can kill you!

'Live hard, die young and have a good looking corpse,' was a saying that did the rounds when I was a young journalist, mainly because that is indeed what journalists did. We drank, we smoked, we worked long hours and were stressed and many of us did die younger than many other professions. We thought it was funny at the time, but this section is not about racing towards the grave and looking as good as you can – in fact it's about how you can avoid your skin being the reason that you end up in a grave before your time.

One look in the mirror as we age will let us know that our skin loses elasticity and firmness, that fine lines and wrinkles begin to show and over time it can start to look dry and more crepe-like. In fact, studies show that our skin loses about 30 per cent of its collagen in the first five years after menopause. After that, it starts to slow and we lose about 2 per cent every year for the next 20 years.[13]

Aesthetically that may not be fun, and I'll deal with that shortly, but first, there's a darker side we need to deal with. We may start to notice that the thinner skin on our bodies bruises more easily. That's because from about 55–60 years of age onwards we start to head towards what's known as skin fragility – thin crepe-like skin on our bodies. We may notice that those little bruises start to turn into purple blotches called senile purpura. And we may also notice that all those little cuts and bruises take longer to heal. I don't want to be a killjoy here, but much like bladder infections, this can be a killer.

London-based consultant dermatologist Dr Clare Kiely emphasises that skin fragility is a serious health risk for older adults. 'When the skin takes longer to heal, the risk of infections like cellulitis increases, and if untreated, this can develop into sepsis, which can be "life-threatening",' she explains.[14] Dermatoporosis is the relatively new term for it, first coined in 2007[15] and she says it often affects the forearms and lower legs, the areas that are frequently exposed to the sun and damaged as a result and are also more prone to injury from knocks and bumps as we move around.

With an ageing population this is going to be an increasingly important issue according to Dr Angela Tewari, who is also a consultant dermatologist in London. 'The term skin fragility in dermatology originally refers to skin fragility disorders as a group of conditions in which the structural integrity of the skin is compromised and its resistance to external shear forces are diminished.' And collagen plays a big part in the structural integrity. Tewari says there are various types of collagen that make up what's called our extracellular matrix (the structures that give our skin firmness and resilience) including types 1, 3 and 7. With age and declining oestrogen levels these reduce, as does elastin which gives our skin its spring. There's also an effect on the integrity of blood vessels in the skin – without a good framework supporting them they don't withstand pressure and trauma in the same way they used to, and that's why we bruise and tear more easily.

How to maintain skin strength as you age

So, what can be done to support ageing skin on your body and reduce fragility? According to Dr Kiely these key strategies can help:

- Prioritise a nutrient-rich diet – eat plenty of polyphenols and antioxidants from fruits and vegetables, and ensure you get an adequate amount of protein in your diet to support collagen synthesis.
- Use a high-quality moisturiser – choose one with hyaluronic acid, ceramides and niacinamide and vitamin C (L-ascorbic acid in at least a 5 per cent concentration) to hydrate and strengthen the skin barrier. Basically – treat your body with the same care as your face.
- Stay well-hydrated – proper hydration helps maintains skin elasticity and barrier function.
- Avoid smoking and excessive alcohol – both inhibit collagen production, accelerating skin thinning.
- Protect yourself against sun damage. 'The sun is the enemy of collagen,' says Dr Kiely. Use a broad-spectrum sunscreen that blocks UVA and UVB rays, and if possible, cover your skin with clothing to minimise exposure. 'We don't tend to see this kind of damage in skin that hasn't been exposed to the sun.'

Advanced skincare interventions

For those looking to further protect and improve skin resilience, Dr Kiely suggests incorporating topical treatments backed by research:

- Retinoids (Vitamin A) – these stimulate collagen renewal and may help strengthen fragile skin, but can irritate. There are now body moisturisers available with added retinol.
- Synthetic Vitamin D (Calcitriol/Calcipotriol) – an emerging treatment showing promise in slowing skin thinning and supporting epidermal integrity, only available on prescription.

By taking proactive steps to look after our skin, she says, we can reduce fragility, lower the risk of infections and ensure that ageing skin remains healthy, resilient and better protected against damage. When it comes to the face or body in general, Dr Mandy Leonhardt, menopause GP and author of *What Every Woman Needs to Know about Their Skin and Hair*, says: 'You do not need to soap your whole body, soaps are usually alkaline and they can strip the protective oils off your skin; a pH neutral shower oil or gel is more gentle. If you're a lover of baths, avoid bubble baths as they can dry out your skin too much. Add some bath oil or magnesium flakes instead.'

Another tip she says is applying your body moisturiser on damp skin. 'Just pat it dry after bathing and apply a thick layer and let it soak in.' When it comes to cleansing, she recommends an oil-based or creamy cleanser for the face. We tend to over cleanse, she says, and this can irritate the skin.

The skin–bone axis

You may have noticed skin and bone have things in common, among them is collagen, and there's a growing school of thought that's looking at what's called the 'skin–bone axis'.[16] It goes along the lines of this: the skin can be a mirror of our health, reflecting many of the diseases of the internal organs. An example of this is dry skin for hypothyroid conditions or jaundice (yellow skin) in liver disease. Even though there are obvious differences between soft tissues like skin and solid bones, they are closely related. Both consist of fibroblasts and osteoblasts which are involved in the production of collagen – the scaffolding of bone and skin. How much collagen we have and how good its quality is can be affected by ageing, declining oestrogen levels, diseases like diabetes and inflammation as well as certain medications like glucocorticoids. These similarities have led researchers to look more closely at what they call the 'crosstalk' between them for ways that they can diagnose and treat conditions like osteoporosis in the future. So, cutting a long story short – your skin could be an indicator for the condition of your bones.

Dr Leonhardt says this relationship between the bone and skin has been around since the 1930s and says if your skin is extremely frail, for example it breaks easily and doesn't heal quickly or if it comes off when you remove a Band-Aid or plaster, then ask your doctor about having a DEXA scan to see what your bone mineral density is. 'It's pain free, very safe and quite cheap if you can't get one on the NHS.' Knowing your bone mineral density can help you manage your future fracture risk.

Boobs and bras – why can't I wear my bra anymore?

This is a hugely common problem and I faced it myself. As things started to head south and a bit of extra weight went on, I started to notice that my bra was becoming increasingly uncomfortable. I could hardly wear it and couldn't wait to get it off at the end of the day. For a while all I could wear was sports bras as everything else felt like it was rubbing the skin under my boobs raw. It took me a while to put two and two together but it slowly dawned on me that sweat could be the problem. There wasn't any redness under the breasts or anything that screamed fungal infection but I thought I'd take a proactive step. I had a chat with a dermatologist and I started to use an antifungal. I tightened my bra straps up to make sure there was less skin rubbing, washed my towels more frequently in hot water and within six weeks or so the skin was much happier. If this sounds like you, get the skin under your breasts checked, and see if this might be an appropriate course of action for you. The condition is called interigo and general advice for dealing with it includes:

- Wash under your breasts morning and night with a gentle soap or soap substitute (for example emulsifying ointment). This is especially important after exercising.

- Dry the area thoroughly – gently pat dry with a clean, soft towel. Some people find a hairdryer on a cool setting works well if the skin is super sensitive.
- Wash towels regularly and don't share them to avoid spreading infection.
- Get a well-fitting, supportive bra made from a natural material such as cotton. (Synthetic fabrics can be a sweat trap.)
- Try to maintain a healthy weight – so there's less skin on skin, so to speak.

A biting question – gum disease and tooth loss

Just like your skin, your gums can be an indicator of your internal health too. Gum disease has been associated with an increased risk of blood vessel issues and heart disease.[17] This may be because it may induce inflammation in the blood vessels. It's not a cause of heart disease, but an association. But, if you've got gum disease – don't ignore it. We know postmenopausal women are at increased risk of tooth loss for a variety of reasons, but it too has been associated with poor bone health.[18] There have been suggestions that MHT may help with preventing tooth loss and gum disease – but nothing beats basic dental hygiene. And recently a study suggested that regular flossing could decrease the risk of stroke[19] – so there's another incentive to take that wax strip to those pearly whites!

Tips for tooth and gum health

- Brush twice a day and floss daily.
- Avoid smoking – it can cause gum disease as it constricts blood flow, but it can also mask it as you won't bleed as much.
- Remember foods like fruit and carbonated drinks including sparkling water are a mild acid and can affect tooth enamel too, so brush after those.
- See your dentist/dental hygienist at least once a year (twice is better).
- Limit sugary foods.

Menopause can cause a dry mouth and without enough saliva, bacteria can build up on the teeth and gum line and increase the risk of tooth loss. Try sipping water regularly through the day, chewing gum (beware if it's the sugar-free type though as it may see you running to the toilet) or you can get artificial saliva from your chemist. Limiting caffeine and alcohol can help too as they're dehydrating, as is smoking. Try a humidifier at night.[20]

Musculoskeletal syndrome of menopause

Are your muscles and joints aching? Got a frozen shoulder? Are your muscles wasting away? It could be the musculoskeletal syndrome of menopause. This is a new term that's hit the medical journals recently which was put forward by Dr Vonda Wright and colleagues.[21] She's an orthopaedic surgeon in the US and over the years she and her colleagues have noticed that women around the time of menopause were consistently showing up with similar conditions and complaints that were affecting their quality of life. Like the Genitourinary Syndrome of Menopause (GSM) they argue that the thing in common here is declining oestrogen and that these conditions, which include pain in the muscles, bones and joints, loss of muscle mass, loss of bone density leading to osteoporosis and increased fracture risk, tendon and ligament injuries, adhesive capsulitis (frozen shoulder) and cartilage matrix fragility, or the breakdown of cartilage which may lead to osteoarthritis, should be regarded as a syndrome too.

In many ways, it makes sense and they've urged the title to be embraced by the menopause community. As for treatments, they suggest:

- A healthy diet with adequate vitamin and mineral intake such as vitamin D and K2
- MHT if appropriate
- Appropriate exercise.

I know it seems counterintuitive to keep on moving if you're in pain but it is important. It's a good idea if you find it painful or have injuries to visit a physiotherapist as they can advise you about which stretches or exercises are best for you. If you are in the UK you can self-refer via the NHS and it's free.

4

WHY IT MATTERS – POLITICS, POWER AND BEING YOUR OWN ADVOCATE

When the world is silent, even one voice becomes powerful.

– Malala Yousafzai

11

Power to the people

In 1918, the first woman was elected to parliament in the UK. Her name was Constance Markievicz but since she represented Sinn Fein, the Irish Republican Party, she wasn't allowed to take up her seat. That election also marked the first time a select group of women – those over 30 who owned property – were allowed to vote. We're now coming up to the centenary of all women over the age of 21 being afforded that privilege, but how far have we really come in terms of making our presence felt in the hallowed corridors of power? As of July 2024, women held 263 out of the 650 seats in parliament, or about 40 per cent, but when it comes to cabinet posts over the 20 years to 2024 we've held on average just 22 per cent.[1] In boardrooms we only hold 25.8 per cent of executive directorships and 9 per cent of board-room chairs. This is a vast improvement though from 2019 when it was just 4.2 per cent.[2] So, it's fair to say we still have a long way to go to achieve parity, even though, according to a McKinsey report, gender diversity in the boardroom contributes an extra 25 per cent profitability to companies – and ethnic diversity makes it even better at 36 per cent.[3] So surely it would make sense to remove any barriers to inclusion from the start to finish of every woman's working life?

Unfortunately, history shows us that overcoming the barriers that affect our ability to achieve parity, let alone stay in work and climb the greasy pole in the first place, have been hard-won battles and are still ongoing. Let's take a look at maternity leave. It was introduced in the UK in 1975 for women who had been employed for two years, but it wasn't until 1993 that all women were entitled to it, regardless of how long they'd been employed. This brought the UK in line with the EU. In the US maternity leave was only made available in 1993 under the Temporary Disability Act. It allowed for 12 weeks of unpaid leave, but not for everyone. It depends on the size of the company you work for and how long you've worked there. The US is still the only OECD country that doesn't have a national system of paid maternity leave, with each state currently overseeing its own programme. This puts it on a par with a handful of countries – seven, in fact – that still have no national maternity leave programmes. Most of those are small Pacific Islands.

While government employees in Australia had the benefit of maternity leave from 1973, the rest of the nation's working women had to wait until 2011 for the Paid Parental Leave Act 2010 to be enacted. It allowed for 18 weeks of paid leave at the minimum wage. Prior to that, if you worked in the private sector, it was determined by your employment contract, or was taken as unpaid leave, or covered by accumulated holiday or long service leave payments.

Once your leave is finished (if you get it at all), you may want to return to work and you will most likely need childcare, but you will quickly find that access to affordable options is almost impossible, even in the richest of countries, because the allowances paid don't come close to meeting the costs. For low to middle income earners the cost of childcare is often prohibitive, with a report in the UK, aptly titled 'Pregnant then Screwed', showing that three-quarters (76 per cent) of mothers paying for childcare said it no longer made financial sense for them to continue to work.[4] Some 26 per cent said it now costs them more than 75 per cent of their take-home pay, and a third (32 per cent) said they had to rely on some form of debt to cover their childcare bills. Given we know the economic benefits of having women in the workplace, that's hardly an incentive to return, so you would think that adequate maternity leave and childcare support would be no brainers. But they have constantly been met with resistance because of the cost to business or the taxpayer. The result?

- Women have to and continue to bear the economic loss in terms of income, savings, future pension or the superannuation benefits that we discussed in Chapter 5.
- They've also had to battle discrimination because employers were wary of giving women of child-bearing age a job for fear they'd immediately get pregnant and became a spreadsheet liability, or if they were already in work they'd be sacked or demoted to reduce costs to the employer. In the end, laws like the 2010 Equality Act in the UK were introduced to stop these kinds of practices – some 17 years after access to maternity leave was expanded.[5]

Now it's the turn of menopause in the policy spotlight – and again it's controversial because it rattles the perception of what women should be like at work. It was bad enough that we had periods and then babies, but now we're bleeding everywhere all the time, moody, irrational and can't even do our jobs properly anymore! And as we wade through this morass in a hot sticky mess, we enter a whole new world – the world of gendered ageism.

There is some amazing work being done on this in academic circles, so let me give you a quick insight into some of it, summarised succinctly by Belinda Steffan and Wendy Loretto at the University of Edinburgh.[6] They've compiled a body of work from current literature looking at 'the ideal worker', showing how menopausal women appear to be the direct opposite of that. A woman's body should not be 'inconvenient or uncomfortable for others' – but menopausal women are. They cite studies showing that as 'experiences of menopause are "brought directly into work," negative gendered-ageist judgments (e.g., disgust and [perceptions of] low commitment) are dependent upon the extent to which the menopausal body is in opposition to ideal worker norms of being, like men, reliable, unemotional and unencumbered'. To avoid that, a menopausal woman who 'takes control of her symptoms' is less likely to breach ideal worker stereotypes and run into trouble. But a steadily growing number of women are finding themselves in exactly that position – trouble.

Back in late 2018 Maria Rooney, a child social worker in Leicestershire, resigned because she felt she had been treated unfairly due to the impact of her menopause symptoms, anxiety and depression, on her ability to work. In January 2019, with the support of the Equality and Human Rights Commission (EHRC), she lodged claims with the Employment Tribunal against Leicester City Council and was successful.[7] Writing about the case, the EHRC said the Employment Tribunal 'decided that Ms Rooney was disabled at all material times covered by her claims. It ruled that Ms Rooney's disability was by virtue of her symptoms of menopause combined with symptoms of stress and anxiety.' It was the first Employment Appeal Tribunal decision to conclude that menopause symptoms can amount to a disability for the purposes of the Equality Act 2010, and it set a legal precedent – that she was discriminated against on the grounds of disability and sex.

Since Rooney's case there have been a growing number of cases heading to tribunals. In 2020 there were 16 cases brought, and that jumped to 23 in 2021. In 2022 it dipped to 18 cases, but the first six months alone of 2023 saw 14. And there have been some hefty payouts awarded, with one woman receiving just over £64,000 after the tribunal ruled that her employer had refused to make reasonable adjustments for her.[8]

As the number of cases grew, so too did calls for menopause to be included as a 'protected characteristic' under the Equality Act. This would mean categorising menopause symptoms that affect work as a 'disability' – but it's not a word that's embraced by all. Arguments raged in opinion pieces and articles across the press, raising fears that it would be yet another way to make women unemployable.

Mariella Frostrup, menopause advocate, co-founder of Menopause Mandate and the second menopause workplace ambassador articulated this stance well in *The Times*, saying: 'We've campaigned really hard for what's a perfectly natural life stage not to be considered a disability. I think this feels in many ways like a step backwards. Menopause is not a disability, it's a staging post of women's fertility journey that like all the others from puberty onwards needs to be factored in to how we create a modern workplace. At every stage . . . women are penalised in the workplace, particularly economically for their unique biology. We need to be thinking about full scale reshaping of our workplace.'

Kent University's organisational psychologist, Hannah Swift, agrees the terminology could be damaging to women. 'I think there is a danger because you're reinforcing a narrative of incompetence. We've been trying to fight this idea, saying we have parity, and that we're not typically seen as less competent than men. And now suddenly we're saying, "oh, actually, when you reach a certain age, or when this happens to you, you are going to experience some things which do make you less competent". So, it's really tricky narrative to have, and I think it needs to be framed in a way that it's not about competence.'

Ultimately the government rejected calls to make menopause a protected characteristic under the Act, but if a person's symptoms are seen to be impacting on their ability to perform it could be considered a disability and if they are penalised for it, or reasonable adjustments to accommodate them aren't taken by their employer, the employee can take action against them.[9] Additionally, an employer cannot discriminate against you on the grounds of gender, gender reassignment, and they cannot make comments against you that are seen as ridiculing or belittling your symptoms as that would be harassment.

What are some examples of reasonable adjustments?

Where possible allowing for:

- flexible working hours
- adjusting uniform requirements to allow for cooler clothes
- providing rest areas or cooler areas where staff can sit
- providing fans
- easy access to bathrooms.

These don't have to cost a lot and the EHRC points out these kinds of adjustments could be far less costly than a big pay out, legal fees and the cost of replacing staff if they resign.[10]

But is the word 'disability' a red herring? Weiss-Wolf isn't that hung up on it. 'Do we need to really change the words? Maybe, but I mean, on the other hand, there's a lot to learn from the disability community and how it's been advocating, the kinds of reforms that it's championed, especially since the pandemic. When we think about the workplace, we've actually as a society created a workplace that that is a whole lot friendlier and much more flexible to the way people with disabilities might need to operate.'

Semantics aside, women in the UK should consider themselves lucky, because Weiss-Wolf says there are virtually no protections for menopausal women in the US at present, so her focus for change will be looking at pregnancy regulations.

'There's very little federal menstrual legislation that's been passed in this country and the only federal menstrual legislation that we have was signed by President Donald Trump when he was president the first time around. So, it is true that randomly good things can slide in. We don't need to have a big banner, all lights flashing "menopause law" passed, but all that stuff can get written into other research bills or other bills that have to do with health care or research or education or employment. This stuff is now fodder for a lot of different potential opportunities.'

At the moment though 'we have no framework, really, for protection. The only place that menopause shows up, even tangentially, is in something called the Pregnant Workers Fairness Act', a more modern version of which is the Pregnancy Discrimination Act. She says there have been inferences, that because it references menstruation and discrimination, it could be a place to address menopause discrimination. Other acts, like the Americans with Disabilities Act, have been mentioned too but none of them are anywhere near 'the bottom line or the end game which means when we talk about menopause in the workplace, there is no guarantee against discrimination on the basis of menopause. So, while you might be debating over whether disability is the right framework, especially when menopause is a normal stage of life, not necessarily something one would qualify as an exception, like a disability, at least there's something. There's actually nothing here other than trying to interpret discrimination on those three bases.'

With all her experience in lobbying for changes to laws governing tampon taxes Weiss-Wolf was hoping changes to legislation around menopause would follow a similar path but she quickly discovered it wasn't going to be that easy.

'It's so interesting because I thought when I went into this that I had the whole playbook and I just had to reset it a little bit for menopausal people, and that's not true at all. Menstruation related stuff, the quality of the legislation is quite different. Making menstrual products more affordable or available, or even thinking about the safety of menstrual products, all of that doesn't require the same investment in science and research and much more sophisticated interventions as menopause. So that's where it's different.'

But she's hoping that some areas of similarity might prove to be its strength. 'They both avoid some of the partisan politicking and can stay out of the fray on things that are more contentious or more challenging to advance. Another area, she says, is capitalising on the draft legislation that exists as well as other elements that have made it into other bills when you weren't expecting to see advances. 'I'm hoping we can do some of the same this time for menopause.'

Processes and transparency – did I forget to mention my conflict of interest?

While she's pondering the legislative quandaries, the corridors of power in both hemispheres are busy places with lobby groups, company representatives and individuals all trying to get their particular interests recognised. It's a common and perfectly legal practice. So, it's probably not surprising that the pharmaceutical companies who've seen the upsurge in prescribing in the UK over the past few years would like to see a similar 'Davina effect' down under. Both countries have similar 'universal care' health systems, but Australia's Pharmaceutical Benefits Scheme (PBS), which subsidises the cost of medicines to make them affordable, doesn't, at the time of writing, have as many MHT options on it as the UK does. (They do, however, have a testosterone cream specifically for women, but it is not yet available on the PBS so is quite costly.)

In 2024 the Australian Senate, or 'upper house', held an inquiry into menopause that took around 400 verbal and written submissions from a variety of individuals, healthcare providers, researchers, industry bodies and various pharmaceutical companies. Professor Samantha Thomas and her colleagues analysed the submission for declarations of conflicts of interest[11] and found that only three of the 284 written submissions (1 per cent) mentioned anything about conflicts of interest. They were from Monash University, the Jean Hailes Foundation (an Australian women's health charity) and the Australasian Menopause Society. Out of the 126 verbal submission, just ten people (6 per cent) declared a conflict of interest. Overall, that's a declaration rate of just 3.17 per cent.

Some of those who gave submissions had received payments from pharmaceutical companies that manufacture MHT in the recent past for previous submissions they had worked on for other areas of government or for their work as healthcare professionals delivering, for example, menopause education to other practitioners, as is standard practice. Others were providers of private menopause health services or workplace programmes, both of which would benefit from recommendations that would improve access to or support their businesses. Some had a foot in all four of those camps. And there were submissions from the manufacturers of MHT too, including Besins and Theramex.

Individuals who made submissions may argue that they hadn't received payments for this particular inquiry so a declaration wasn't relevant, but Thomas argues if they had in the past, it should have been declared, and if they had businesses interests that could benefit, that too should have been made clear as it is relevant.

Does it matter if they didn't? Thomas argues that transparency is hugely important. Declaring a conflict of interest won't make it go away but at least you can evaluate the information given if you have that knowledge. A good example of this is a study done by the manufacturer of a product which finds its product is amazing. Would you give it the same weight as an independent evaluation? No, you would weigh the independent study higher as you'd expect the manufacturer to say their product is the best. In this case though, Thomas says, it just didn't happen. Declarations were asked for at the start of the day in the oral sessions, but the call was not repeated so those who arrived later may not have known they should be declaring any conflicts of interest. Individual members of the public may not be aware they need to declare conflicts of interests but those who work in the industry should know, she says.

'There was a failure at every step of the way with that and it has huge ramifications for the development of policy. It's really important because of the need to protect women's health from vested interests, and if we don't have systematic processes, not only to ensure transparency around conflicts of interest, but also how they are then dealt with in making policy recommendations, it's incredibly problematic for women's health . . . We end up with recommendations, but we don't know essentially what has influenced those recommendations.'

While it might be obvious that pharma companies have a conflict of interest as they potentially stand to benefit from recommendations that expand the prescribing options, she wonders why they were at the inquiry in the first place. 'If we were having an inquiry into the tobacco industry, the tobacco industry would not be allowed a seat at the table. So why, when we have something as precious as women's health, are we not being as thorough and as rigorous around potential commercial interests influencing the evidence that's given and the decisions that are made?'

Vikram Talaulikar couldn't agree more. 'They should not be anywhere near it, 100 per cent. Pharmaceutical agents or companies should be nowhere near anybody who is in the deciding chair about making policies for helping menopausal women. It's a catastrophe. You've got to get people who are neutral, who have no connections with pharma.' His concern extends to healthcare professionals who have been paid to deliver education by pharmaceutical companies in the past too. Their declaration has to clearly mention the sponsorship or any honorarium received for this event or in the past.

'There is always conflict of interest. There is always a subconscious bias that goes into what you present and you should not submit anything.' In an ideal world he'd like to see all funded submissions declared and removed otherwise he fears 'it's a complete whitewash'. These may be utopian views, but at least if conflicts past and present are known the appropriate weight can be given to the information provided.

In the end, the pharma companies did indeed benefit from the inquiry with the government recommending that three new hormone replacement drugs be added to the PBS, giving Australian women more options at an affordable price. So that's a good thing.

But, how did the inquiry come about in the first place? In November 2024, a podcast went to air called 'Dear Menopause'. In it, the host, an Australian menopause advocate, discussed the process with her friend, another menopause advocate called Johanna Wicks. Wicks described how she was employed by a pharmaceutical company to lobby for greater menopause awareness within political circles. She didn't mention the name of the company but said: 'There was absolutely no discussion about, you know, increasing any kind of product sales. It was very much about "we see that women in Australia don't know very much about menopause and perimenopause"' and what could be done to change that. Wicks then described how she went away and looked at the list of female politicians and approached those who she thought would be around perimenopause/menopause and after various visits to Canberra and events hosted, an inquiry was born. The host of the podcast said Wicks is '99% responsible' for bringing it to fruition.[12] It turns out that the company was Besins. In a 2025 interview with *The Guardian* Wicks said she had always been open about this and a spokesperson for Greens senator Larissa Waters, who took up the cause to get the inquiry off the ground after Wick's lobbying, said she had always been clear that she was working for Besins.[13] But it may not have been that clear to the public. The Senate's recommendations and the government's response do not state anywhere that the inquiry was brought about by pharma company lobbying.

'In a democracy we would expect that there would be full disclosures, not only around why the inquiry was set up and how it was set up, but also from those testifying or submitting evidence to the inquiry, and then also on how politicians had then managed and considered that evidence moving forward,' Thomas says.

But, I hear you say, does this really matter? As long as women get what they need and have their lived experience recognised after so many centuries of, well, crap, then where's the harm? Surely the means justify the end, which is the betterment of women's health? And surely those who criticise the lack of disclosure are being 'anti-women'? Well, Thomas argues, it does matter, because you can't protect women's health if you don't have robust and open processes in place.

'I would say this position is "pro women", because what we're trying to do is to protect women from exploitation. And you know, we have seen this before with other industries, and there are very significant concerns around the very big commercial market opportunities relating to menopause, not just from the pharmaceutical industry, but also from private clinics and from the wellness industry. And we know the vulnerability of women's health issues to corporate capture. So, this is saying we need to be doing as much as possible to make sure that women get evidence-based care and treatment that are accessible and affordable for them, and that the systems are there to serve the best interests of women's health, not the best interests of companies that are trying to make profit from them.'

And it's not just exploitation or business gains – there's a bigger picture here. If you substitute 'contraception' for 'menopause' and the lobbyist for example, a pro-life organisation, you may not be so happy with the outcome (depending on which side of the fence you site on that particular debate).

If you think the UK is immune to this kind of lobbying from pharma, which is of course perfectly legal and common practice, you'd be wrong. The All Party Parliamentary Group (APPG) on menopause received around £125,000 from Theramex, Astellas, Bayer and Bristol Myers Squibb between 2021 and 2023 via international advisory groups acting as the APPG's secretariat.[14,15,16]

The money, around £5,000/month, was used for social media, a website and other expenses related to the running of the group. To give you a guide on what the secretariats do, another company that provides these services to other APPGs says, 'As the secretariat, we are responsible for the day to day running of these groups and help bring together interested parties, produce reports and host events, among other activities.'

If you want to check and see if a practitioner has received funding from a pharmaceutical company most countries will have a searchable database. In the UK it's Disclosure UK, in the US it's Open Data, and in Australia it's Disclosure Australia. Disclosure UK also gives links to pharma company websites where they show how much they've spent on payments to members of the public, journalists, social media campaigns and patient groups.

And pharma companies are quite active when it comes to supporting UK patient groups. A 2020 study shows 1,422 payments were made by 74 pharma companies to 341 patient organisations. And while you may be thinking this is purely philanthropic they found that 'almost all funds (90%) from pharmaceutical companies were directed to patient organisations that are aligned with companies' approved drug portfolios and research and development pipelines'.[17]

To Moynihan these are classic pharma tactics: 'Creating the need for a product is one of the basic marketing strategies of the corporations who sell pharmaceuticals', and we need to be more vigilant. 'Everyone should be more aware of how industry uses layers of sophisticated marketing to undermine public debates about health-care. Rather than blindly accept the propaganda – often funnelled through funded "third parties" – we should be investigating and stopping these unhealthy flows of money.'

Other studies show that when these types of things start to happen the patient advocacy groups start to support the products being produced by the companies that are funding them. One shows how patient groups with affiliations to lobby groups urging the US FDA to approve of the 'female viagra' – Flibanserin (a drug for female sexual dysfunction), showed remarkable similarities in what they said in their submissions – it's a 'severe medical condition' that 'no amount of talking therapy is going to fix'. Submissions from groups without affiliations talked more about relationships, psychotherapy and communication.[18] That phrase, 'no amount of talking therapy' may sound familiar if you followed the debate about the controversial draft changes to the 2024 NICE Guidelines on menopause which suggested a greater emphasis on CBT for low mood/depression in menopause. Facebook groups and social media posts were full of comments from women saying they were being fobbed off again, that this was akin to being told their symptoms were 'all in their head' and that 'no amount of talking was going to fix their symptoms' – MHT was and should be the first-line option. In the end the draft guidelines were reworded to make the latter clearer. (CBT for menopause vasomotor symptoms does have good evidence backing it according to the Menopause Society's Non Hormonal Position Statement[19] and can be an effective adjunct to hormone therapy or an alternative for those who cannot or do not wish to take MHT. It doesn't have to be one or the other, it can be both.)

The upshot of this is that people do indeed have a voice, as they absolutely should – but transparency is a must.

Reports and recommendations

Over the past five years there has been endless talking. There have been task forces set up, numerous reports and women's health strategies written and pages and pages of recommendations on how to move forward and ensure menopausal women are best served. There have been wins with a prepayment certificate that has seen the cost for MHT capped at under £20/year in England, two topical vaginal products have made it onto pharmacy shelves that are available without a prescription if you are over 50 and symptomatic. We've had a 'Tsar' appointed to deal with HRT shortages (which are still ongoing globally), two menopause workplace ambassadors, and a women's health ambassador. And we've had £25 million over two years for the establishment of Women's Health Hubs, but not all have menopause services in them and as I write, their future isn't guaranteed.

Among the recommendations made, there have been calls for the 40+ health check to be expanded to include a discussion on menopause, but that is still 'being explored'. In Australia the Senate inquiry recommended a similar move and the Labor government agreed in early 2025 that it would look to see how it best fitted into the current time-based tiers for consultations.

In both countries there were recommendations for a national menopause campaign. The Australian government said yes and allocated AU$12 million for it, but the UK isn't keen, deeming it unnecessary even though multiple surveys of women show time and time again that the menopause world is a bubble and those outside it, especially those in deprived areas or those who come from culturally different backgrounds, have little idea about menopause and are left struggling with their symptoms in isolation. The government claims instead its updated NHS website will do the trick, even though very few people go to websites these days, and if you don't know your symptoms are related to menopause you're hardly likely to go to that page in the first place.

Research has been spoken about as a priority but there's been no extra cash for menopause research in the UK. Instead the publicly funded body that awards payments for research, the National Institute of Health and Care Research (NIRH), was instructed to conduct a 'research prioritisation exercise' to identify research recommendations, and it has, however, allocated funding to a testosterone study, which is good news. In the US the Biden administration did shift money around plus delivered a considerable amount of new funding to menopause but the Trump administration's cuts have dealt a huge blow and almost succeeded in shutting down the

Women's Health Initiative completely. As controversial as aspects of it have been, it is the longest running study of women's health and its insights are invaluable.

Compulsory continued professional development for current medical practitioners has been knocked back in the UK and Australia but the latter has said they will spend some money to incentivise doctors to do menopause training. In the UK, high school and medical students are now receiving some education, so that's a win, and we have a lot of activity in terms of workplace policies, pledges, training programmes or initiatives that will help ensure workers are supported.

For advocates like Jennifer Weiss-Wolf and Diane Danzebrink, if we had those basic blocks in place in terms of good, accessible public information and a well-educated medical workforce, many of these reports would be redundant because women would be getting the support they needed.

But given that isn't our current situation, Weiss-Wolf would like 'every workplace that implements a menopause benefits programme or coaching or HR policy or whatever – I would like to see them tied to it by supporting these broader policies for research and medical education and consumer education. This is where I start.'

For Danzebrink, 'the most frustrating thing is that the solutions to the problems are actually very simple. Number one, the lack of primary care menopause training could easily be resolved with a short CPD training video distributed by the NHS. This could be delivered to the inbox of every primary care medical health practitioner. A time limit of three months could be given for them all to watch the one-hour CPD training video and a clever tech system could record once each practitioner has completed the training. And hey presto! Every single GP, practice nurse or primary care practitioner would be up-to-date with current menopause training, ending the menopause care lottery for patients and helping practitioners feel confident to support those patients make informed choices.

'Number two is you have a public health campaign that runs consistently for at least 12 months to include resources for teachers so they feel that they can confidently teach their students about it. And three: the Department of Work and Pensions, produces a free menopause support resource for all workplaces.

'But this is the thing that really bugs me – none of these things are expensive, the benefit to cost ratio is enormous and they could all be done easily within a 12-month period, and all of that could have been done 10 years ago. But what we end up with is endless meetings about meetings, and more surveys and reports and a 10-year Women's Health Strategy which has absolutely no plan for full implementation. It's all very well having meetings and reports, but we don't need more words, because if all of the words had turned into actions we would be a lot further forward. And I know for many of us who have been campaigning on this subject for many years now, we feel like we are just screaming into the wind.'

Chair of the BMS Janice Rymer agrees doctors need more education and says she and others in the field have been working on a tool for GPs that will make their lives so much easier when it comes to diagnosing and treating menopausal women, but bureaucracy within the NHS has buried it. 'One of my previous jobs in the last three years was the national specialty advisor for NHS England, and we have devised a fantastic tool called "the optimal pathway for GPs". Honestly, it's great, and it's just for exactly that – most GPs do not know a lot about management. It's such a good information source. So, we are trying. But NHS England said, "Oh, we don't know where to put it."'

Moving forward

All of this leads us to ask: Where to next in this period of distrust, confusion and conflict where we have doctors battling it out on social media, slow policy changes and a very confused public?

There needs to be some serious bridge building, but can both sides of the evidence chasm come to a détente to bring the focus back to where it should be – the betterment of women's health. At the moment we have a situation where women are caught in the middle of a confusing set of battles between those who are accused of being out-of-touch gatekeepers of information and those who are said to be promoting theories that aren't currently supported by evidence. Somewhere there must be some common ground especially in terms of education, information and access to affordable service across the globe.

'Again, it's like this big, big pool of twine that has to be like unwound,' says Weiss-Wolf. We approach things with a very black-and-white view but sometimes we may need to accept that two things can be true at the same time. 'That doesn't mean that we throw up our hands, or just let one side or the other win, or just let everybody fight with each other in public. I continue to believe if we just focus on the core policy agenda items, we will direct ourselves in a better path, and we'll get some answers along the way. It doesn't mean it's going to solve everything, but it's going to hopefully enable us to line up behind a different vision too.'

What are some of the areas of common ground we could start with?

1 *Updating MHT warnings on prescription product information leaflets:* The removal of outdated information and 'black box' warnings on MHT products is hugely important. If you pick up a vaginal oestrogen product in the UK and US the information inside the box will tell you all of the risks associated with systemic MHT, some of which are outdated or apply to oral or older forms rather than the newer transdermal forms. These include risks of breast, endometrial and ovarian cancers, heart disease and stroke as well as blood clots – none of which are associated with topical vaginal oestrogen but put people off using what is generally regarded as a very safe treatment as a result. Over the past seven years I can't tell you how many women have messaged me to say they are too scared to start using it, let alone the systemic versions. This needs to change. (And by the way, this information at the time of writing is repeated on the NHS website. That's not up-to-date!)

2 *Education for healthcare professionals:* Ensuring all practising primary healthcare doctors, physicians, pharmacists, nurses and nurse pre-scribers, physiotherapists, physicians' assistants and dentists have some basic form of up-to-date medical training on menopause. It doesn't have to be massively time intensive – just enough to ensure they recognise it, understand the basics of the medical and non-medical treatment options and how to find more informa-tion or direct people to where they can find the help they need.

3 *Public health campaigns:* Many menopause advocacy groups have this on their list of things to achieve – but if we all come together maybe we can follow Australia's example in approving a public health campaign and make it a reality. Any information produced should be in multiple languages and multiple formats and available for people across the globe to access.

4 *Improving regulations:* We need these on:
  ○ Unscrupulous claims and treatments. We need to strengthen advertising standards and fact-checking systems (no thanks to Meta here who said they'd be pulling back on fact-checking in the name of free speech).
  ○ Workplace protections to better protect people from harassment, discrimination, age and genderism, and unfair dismissal.

5 *Ring-fencing funding and proactively supporting menopause research:* Being the founder of a charity that supports menopause research, of course I'm going to say this (note the disclosure!) As we know, women's health research in general only attracts around 2 per cent of funding, and in the UK, the amount spent on menopause research by the National Institute of Health and Care Research is about 0.3 per cent. This needs to be increased to at least 3 per cent and ring-fenced for menopause. This doesn't require new money, just a reallocation of existing funds.

6 *Ensuring treatment costs are affordable and available globally:* Generic products should be available where appropriate at an affordable price and for newer drugs, subsidies on each country's drug listings should be pushed for.

7 *Ensuring access to treatments when required:* At the moment access to certain forms of MHT in the UK is a postcode lottery and a national formulary is needed so there is equitable access to treatments across the country. In the US it can be a state-by-state or insurance lottery. These inequities need to end, and barrier to access in other countries addressed.

8 *A 40+ and 50+ menopause consultation:* Yes, both! At the moment some countries have a 'midlife check' but they aren't fit for purpose when it comes to peri- or postmenopausal women. In the UK and Australia it tends to be, as the name suggests, in the mid-40s, but it doesn't discuss menopause symptoms and their management, so that's a missed opportunity. While it may look at blood pressure, blood sugar and cholesterol, it may be too early for the changes that happen around the time of menopause, so having a separate one at around 50–51 or when a woman goes through menopause, to talk about those changes that affect long-term health, would help improve our health span. If we don't have

that, we risk having women who get a clean bill of health in their 40s walking away with no idea of the silent changes that could affect them in a few years' time. Two specific consultations could improve women's health, reduce absenteeism and save health systems a lot of money with very little investment. (And, doctors will see less of us 'whining women'!)

9 *Getting an affordable testosterone product for women approved:* If you're anything like me, squeezing a 'pea-sized' dose out of a testosterone sachet made as a single dose for a man every day is hardly a scientific process. My 'peas' range in size from *petits pois* to an edamame bean. (I know there are clever people who've devised all sorts of decanters and syringe systems, but I'm too lazy!) At the moment Australia is the only country that has a product made especially for women, but it's only available privately. It is available privately in the UK too but it costs a lot. Improving access to this or a similar product at an affordable price makes sense, especially as testosterone prescribing rates in the UK have increased 15-fold since 2015 from £150,000's worth to £2.5 million in 2023. That's a big jump. (Of course, much of that prescribing could be to men as the OpenPrescribing statistics don't differentiate by gender.)

10 *Taking a stance against unregulated compounded products and expensive blood and urine tests:* Purveyors of compounded 'bio-identical' hormone replacement products often claim that their products are safer than those made by pharmaceutical companies and 'tailor-made' to your needs. They use the same ingredients as pharmaceutical companies but their products are made by local pharmacies using doses that may not have been studied for safety or efficacy. They are not regulated in the same way as products produced by pharmaceutical companies and may or may not contain what they say they do. They are not supported by any menopause society across the globe. Often providers of these charge huge amounts for blood or urine tests that are repeated regularly. A united stance against these unproven tests and treatments would save women a lot of money and ensure they were getting the treatments that have been shown to be safe and effective.

11 *Calling for health information in newspapers to be taken out from behind paywalls:* One other thing to consider is this. Over the

past decade media organisations have struggled to make money and have put more and more information behind paywalls to try and shore up their coffers. Social media is free, and it has posed a huge challenge to mainstream media who have not just lost revenue but audience too, as people now get their information from TikTok or other social media sites where the algorithm feeds them a diet of what they like to see. This means people are no longer seeing a broad range of views from what are meant to be independent, fair and balanced reporting sources. While this is obviously hugely important for politics and democracy in general, it's also important for receiving balanced information on health issues. So, getting health information out from behind a paywall is vital. Media organisations aren't charities so this will be a challenge, but many still have considerable profits and are also getting money from native advertising, traffic exchanges and sponsored content. By making more information available freely they could then offer more in-depth content, specials or analysis on subscription. At least then the basic information would be out there for all to see, and it could drive traffic to their sites, improve their bounce rates, which would enhance their value to advertisers, and even boost their subscription base.

12 *Ensuring medical journals publish 'plain language' commentaries to explain studies:* The democratisation of medical information has been great, but access to studies will often involve an abstract only unless you pay for the full text, or if it is available to read in full it may not be easy for lay people or the press to understand. A lot of confusion could be avoided if they also published a plain language commentary that explains the findings and their practical implications. With more studies being discussed online this is a very simple thing to do that could help reduce misunderstanding and stop data from being cherry-picked or taken out of context.

These are just a handful of areas where we could come together and lobby to improve women's health and help restore trust. None of these things will happen overnight. We all need to step up and pressure the powers that be to make the changes we need. We need to be in the forefront of MPs' minds, not just a handful of lobbyists. Our voices need to be heard. How do we do that? Backing campaigns, signing petitions, writing to your local politicians or, if you're in the UK, going to one of your MP's 'surgeries' to talk about the issues that concern you. You've made your vote count, now make your voice heard.

As the MP Carolyn Harris said back in June 2022, 'The time for warm words and gestures has well and truly passed. We cannot let menopausal women today suffer any longer, and we must ensure that future generations do not suffer the same experiences as those who came before them. We need a commitment that this will be a priority, and a promise that it will be taken seriously. We need action, and we need it now,'[20] because we still have a long way to go.

12

The good menopause – Put your own mask on first

The last phase is the most glorious.
> – *Dame Julie Walters as Annie in* Calendar Girls *(2003)*

During the reception at my son's wedding a woman in her late 30s came over and told me she watched my Instagram interviews and asked me if there were any good things about menopause. I reeled off the (quite short) list of general benefits – no more periods and period-related symptoms like pain, headaches or PMS, not having to worry about getting pregnant, some say greater self-confidence and not caring as much about what other people think (although I don't really know if either of those are true) and, if you have fibroids – they should shrink.

She folded her arms, looked at me blankly and said: 'Is that it?' Clearly, I hadn't sold it well. None of these were an issue for her, so it didn't really look like a big win. I thought for a few seconds and thought, she's probably right – unless your menstrual life has been hell, the end of it doesn't really sound much like you've finally found the holy grail. But there are indeed pluses.

Georgia University historian and author Susan Mattern says menopause is our superpower. It 'makes us a super adaptable unique species' and even though we may not hold the same status and power in the family unit today as we may have in the past, 'we've gained status in other ways, . . . through business and the workplace'.[1]

Psychologist Hannah Swift agrees – and if it's any consolation, she says some work emerging from the US shows that women who have managed to climb to the top of the corporate ladder actually face less pressure to vacate their seat and make room for the next generation than their male counterparts. It's called the 'intersectional escape hypothesis'.[2] Swift says the basic idea is that women were generally regarded as less competent until they reach a certain position and therefore less of a threat, whereas men are looked at as holding on to power and refusing to step aside and make way for those following in their footsteps. 'It's like women can get away with a bit more because they were never supposed to be there in the first place. Older men are still seen as more threatening to younger people because they're still in those higher positions. You want them to step aside. Women, however, once they reached a certain position, weren't evaluated as negatively as the older male leaders were.'

No matter where we are in our lives, many people find menopause is a time for re-evaluation. Some take a leap and make significant career changes – often for the better. Let's take Kate Oakley, who we met earlier. She was a successful HR specialist, but no longer found her job as fulfilling as she had before, so she retrained to be a personal trainer, and (despite the odd bit of online abuse, as we've seen) she couldn't be happier with her decision. She's found her calling.

Karen Arthur, the founder of Menopause Whilst Black, did a similar thing. After 28 years in teaching, a confluence of life events including menopause and a diagnosis of anxiety and depression made her realise something had to change. As her website explains: 'After a long and difficult journey inwards, she emerged not only happier and healthier, but with a story to share and a mission to follow. Karen took a leap of faith to honour her first love of sewing and fashion by launching a bespoke clothing service that aimed to empower women in their bodies with clothing that made them feel good and stand taller.' She, too, had found her calling and now advocates for women's health and equity as well.

Even though we are the sandwich generation – juggling aging parents, kids at home or still dependent, as well as work, we have a wealth of experience that we can channel into the things we enjoy like hobbies or whole new careers. Business trends in the US show Gen X and Baby boomers are a growing force in establishing new businesses.[3]

So, there is life after menopause, and getting this message across is something Professor Joyce Harper is passionate about.

Professor Harper, a University College London (UCL) reproductive health expert, author, avid cold water swimmer and afternoon raver, has been investigating the positive side of menopause for an upcoming book. She's done in-depth interviews with 51 women about their menopause and how they've emerged 'on the other side' and has found that the 'second spring' can indeed be a good and happy place.

This isn't to say that all the women she spoke to sailed through menopause, in fact she said only a handful did. The rest really had a tough time with some even contemplating suicide. But now, they were 'loving their lives', and in a world where we often focus on the negatives Harper wants to make sure their voices are heard, because they show there can be a light at the end of the tunnel. Describing her own experience she says: 'I definitely felt postmenopause that a cloud had lifted off my brain, and I did have some symptoms – it wasn't plain sailing for me and I did some things to try and help me get through that. But I really felt that cloud had lifted, and I felt such clarity. I felt so strong, and I felt really fabulous, and I felt very much that this was one of the best, if not the best, stage of my life. But I wanted to hear what other women thought, to hear their voices.'

And, without wishing to cannabalise her upcoming book completely (consider this a preview of brilliance to come) what they said was 'they feel now that they are their authentic self. They felt before that they were always doing things for other people, and always felt that they had to act in a particular way and do certain things to please other people and look after other people. And now, they honestly felt that this was the best time of their life. They were really, really thriving. They weren't just surviving.'

What was their trick? It wasn't a miracle cure, a pill or a supplement. It was really back to basics – or as Harper calls them – the five pillars of health:

- Diet
- Exercise
- Sleep
- Mental health
- Friendship and community.

'All of them have really been looking after their lifestyle. They're not all perfect women but the women I interviewed have really got improvements in almost all of those pillars, although quite a few of them are still struggling with sleep. Not all of them exercised but they all did a lot of movement through the day, and they were all eating well, and lots of them have given up alcohol, or really cut back on alcohol, because it doesn't agree with them anymore. So, what they have done is they've listened to their body, they've worked on their body. They've listened to their body, and thought, "What's it saying? Okay, I'm drinking this alcohol. I feel terrible. Okay, stop drinking alcohol. What can help me sleep? Okay, exercise."'

Finding a form of exercise you like is important or you won't stick with it. 'I think we need to find something that brings us joy. Some people love Pilates. I hate Pilates. I told my teacher that day, I do come, but I don't enjoy it, and we should do things that bring us joy.'

Harper's preferred 'torture' (as I call it) is cold water or 'wild' swimming.

'For me, being outside, being in some open water, has always brought me immense pleasure. I always feel it really clears my brain. If I'm upset or anxious or worried it really calms my brain, and my whole body feels incredible. And the euphoria! If you've ever watched me swimming on some of the videos that I've done, I do laugh. I laugh a lot. They say once you get hysterical you should get out, but everyone says "Joyce was hysterical before she got in". There is lots of laughter, if you're with a bunch of middle-aged women, there's also lots of swearing. But you know, we're out in nature. We're with wonderful friends.' And that may be part of the key to it – being in nature, the social connection and having a good laugh – that sense of friendship and community.

Harper has done a bit of preliminary research on this and its relationship with menopause symptoms to try and assess if it made a difference to menopause symptoms. She and her colleagues surveyed 1,114 cold water swimming devotees, 785 of whom were going through the menopause, and found that 46.9 per cent of them experienced an improvement in anxiety, 43.5 per cent in mood swings and 31.1 per cent in low mood, and a further 30.3 per cent in hot flushes – but, as they say, more research is required, and their study is limited by a couple of factors including:

- bias due to the survey being taken by women who already love cold water swimming

- as the survey was conducted online, it is more likely to have been completed by people who noticed an association between menopause symptoms and cold water swimming, skewing the results.[4]

But it's food for thought – if the idea of plunging yourself into icy water appeals. (Personally, I'd rather rip my own ovaries out, but that's just me! If you do decide to give this a go, make sure you have a medical all clear and don't go alone.)

Digital detox

The other thing that Professor Harper says is important is digital downtime. 'Have a digital detox. We're just bombarding ourselves. And lots of the women I've interviewed for my book said the menopause was a wake-up call, even if they were on MHT. We're so stressed. Why are we feeling like that? Is it our body saying: "Hold on, it's all gone a bit crazy, calm down and be still"? Almost every woman said they felt like that when they were in the perimenopause and they wish they'd slowed down a bit more.'

Harper is now trying to have 'silent' days every so often where she doesn't pick up her phone or go on social media. She's also going to meditate more and 'I'm going to go for some walks and just be quiet and be still. I think that's really good for all of us at any stage of our life. Life is hectic, let's just take a breather.'

Put your mask on first

Part of that 'breather' is making time for you – or, in other words, putting your mask on first. This is something I know I fail at miserably, as do many women. We think it's selfish and that we have to look after everyone else first, but sometimes we just need to take some time for ourselves. This was a vital part of Madhu's road to a good menopause after she quit her job, regrouped and started using her HR background to provide workplace support for menopausal women.

'I'm doing something that I passionately love now and I want women to realise that even though you may think there's no light at the end of the tunnel there definitely is,' she says. Asking for help and support from her family was her starting point and she did find it hard, but it made a difference. Then came the lifestyle changes. 'I have had to change everything I eat, my lifestyle, my mindset. I had to prioritise myself. The lesson I've learnt is what they tell you in the safety check on an airplane, "put your own mask on first" – I now understand why they say it. It's because if you have got that mask on, you're looking after your health and your mental health, the people around you are going to be in a much better situation if you're in a good situation. And that's what I feel when it comes to the menopause. If you don't look after yourself, you won't be able to look after everyone else.'

I put the word out to my 'menoposse' on social media to ask people to share what lifestyle changes they'd found helpful and these are some of the answers:

- Exercising more – lifting weights, walking in nature (or anywhere really), yoga, pilates, swimming, cold water swimming
- Mindset – gratitude, focusing on the positive and the things that bring happiness
- Recharging – 'taking time out for me', swapping endless educational podcasts for audiobooks (I can't agree with this more – I never do it, of course, even if I'm in the gym I'm listening to some kind of menopause-related information session! But I do watch a lot of escapist comedies and children's films. My partner finds it very difficult to understand why I no longer prefer a deep and meaningful documentary as I used to – but that's my downtime. No need to think, I have a good laugh and I go to bed happy, not wrecking my brain about how to solve whatever global injustice we've just watched.)
- Making time for joy – dancing, singing, bike riding, friends and family – whatever makes you happy. This was another thing that Harper said was important to the women she interviewed – finding the things that make you happy, no matter how big or small.
- Education – finding good-quality sources of menopause information
- Improving sleep by drinking less alcohol, avoiding caffeine after lunchtime, getting exercise during the day, taking a magnesium supplement at night (I am not advocating that last one as a solution – but was one of the things that popped up repeatedly.)
- Sharing your experience with others and listening to theirs – connecting

- Breathing exercises for relaxation
- Diet – increasing protein and fibre, fruit and veggies, cutting out the highly processed stuff as much as possible
- Reducing stress – going with the flow more, not sweating the little stuff as much

Endocrinology Professor Annice Mukherjee, in her book *The Complete Guide to the Menopause*, says we may need multiple approaches to make the best of our menopause and beyond. The analogy in her book, which I love, is: imagine its winter, you've got a big house and the heaters are on but all the windows are open and you're losing heat. All of the open windows represent the things that are negatively affecting the way you feel, like poor sleep, drinking too much, a poor diet, stress and anxiety. You can focus on shutting one window but you may find that, despite your best efforts, none of the others shut as a result. She gives the example of sleep – you may do everything you can to improve that but you find your anxiety levels haven't changed. So, you're going to have to address all the issues affecting you, which may take time. You don't have to tackle everything at once – but move from room to room. Listen to what your body is telling you, start small, and give yourself time, and slowly more of those windows will start to close and you should start to feel better.

If your diet is poor, you don't have to race to the cupboard, throw out everything in the house and never touch a carb again. Instead many nutritionists and dieticians recommend adding rather than subtracting. Add a piece of fruit to your lunch, add an extra vegetable a day to dinner. Smaller changes are more likely to be sustainable. It's the same with boosting your exercise levels. You don't have to race to the gym and powerlift straight away, or run 5 km. You can start by getting off the bus or the train on the way to work a stop earlier, take the stairs not the lift between floors, go for a walk after dinner, even if it's just around the block, instead of heading straight to the sofa for a Netflix binge. This is what they call 'incidental exercise' and it all adds up. Exercise 'snacks' are becoming increasingly popular – I'm not sure how much evidence there is behind them for changing bone or heart health, as it's early days, but doing something – anything – is better than doing nothing. Examples of these involve things like doing squats while you clean your teeth, or skipping rope, dancing or doing star jumps while the kettle boils – short bursts of activity that at least get you off your bum.

If you haven't exercised for years this sort of activity can start you on the road to getting a bit of strength and fitness back so you can move on to tackle other things later. And don't be embarrassed about starting and not being as fit as others around you. At university I used to run a lot, I never really liked it, but I did it. I even did a half marathon once – it nearly killed me. (I drank way too much water fearing dehydration and sloshed my way slowly from start to finish. The people who did the full marathon finished faster than me.) Over the years, though, with work, travel and a small child, I stopped. In my 40s I thought I needed to start doing some exercise again, so I donned my shorts and runners and took to the pavement. I literally could not run more than the distance between two telegraph poles. So, that's where I started – run one, walk one. The next day I ran two, walked one, and over time that gradually built up to being back at 5 km quite quickly. I didn't care if the neighbours saw me struggling – I was doing it for me.

Like me, some people find exercise classes a daunting prospect. I have no coordination. I could never keep up with step class moves, have fallen off those inflated exercise balls and have had one drop on my face – so I prefer the gym. But in all honesty, I don't think anyone noticed as they were focused on their own moves, and I just laughed. What else can you do? On the upside some people find they make friends in these classes and they can be a social event. If you've never loved exercise, I know you may not believe me, but once you're into a movement groove – even if it feels like hell at the time – you do feel much better afterwards, your mood is improved and you may actually miss it if you don't do it.

If it's stress that's your issue, spend 30 seconds or so looking at something that makes you happy – a flower, a pet, a person, a picture. Practise mindfulness – that clearing of your mind to focus on something other than what's upsetting you. These things can help bring that cortisol level down.

Small changes can build into bigger and better habits over time. And remember, it can be a moveable feast – we change over time, our life stressors and symptoms may change, nothing is static, so we have to be constantly adjusting and tweaking our lifestyles.

Where does all this leave you? Here's a quick recap and some thoughts for the future.

Should you or should you not take MHT?

This is entirely up to you and your healthcare provider. If you have no health reasons to stop you, and your symptoms are worrying you and you think it might help, talk to your doctor about the best options for you. This is *your* body, *your* decision. It is absolutely nobody else's business and their opinions are of zero importance. And if you choose not to – again – 100 per cent *your* decision. Either way, just make sure you are armed with as much information as you can be so you can make an informed choice. If you have vasomotor symptoms it may be worth considering what can bring them under control – and if you don't want, or can't take MHT there are other options now available such as fezolinetant. Sold under the name Veoza in the UK and Veozah in the US, it is a non-hormonal option for treating vasomotor symptoms. Another similar product is elinzanetant. Some low dose antidepressants can help too, and CBT may also be useful.

Should you take MHT as a preventative medicine for your future health?

If you are a midlife woman with no menopause symptoms, the answer at this stage is: no. There is not enough evidence to support taking MHT to prevent dementia, Alzheimer's disease, heart disease or type 2 diabetes – more studies are needed as the consensus is not there when it comes to prevention. As we have mentioned, if your bones are heading towards osteoporosis, or if you went through menopause early or have POI, it's a different story. Talk to your doctor.

Will MHT solve all my problems?

Not necessarily. It can relieve symptoms and for some people it is a 'game changer', literally giving them their life back. But is it going to take every ache away, stop ageing in its tracks and take you back to your 20-year-old self? No. Realistic expectations are important – as is remembering that we are indeed ageing and that some of our symptoms may be related to that or other conditions and those need to be checked out as they arise. And, as every health practitioner will tell you, no amount of MHT can make up for an unhealthy lifestyle.

What about testosterone – is it the missing link that will give me back my energy and clear away those last webs of brain fog?

I know this upsets many people but at the moment, the answer is no. Anecdotally people say it boosts their energy levels and is 'the icing on their MHT cake', but so far, the studies show that it's only effective for improving hyposexual desire disorder (HSDD). That doesn't mean that some people won't find benefits for energy, brain fog and muscle strength, but as yet the studies don't confirm this on big numbers of people; it's not recommended for those things alone. More research is being done as I write and you read.

Is it too late to make lifestyle changes if I'm already in my 50s or beyond?

Hell no! It's never too late to improve your health. Being active, just keeping on moving, helps reduces joint and muscle pain. Being strong and having good balance helps reduce your risk of falling and ending up with a fracture. Eating well can improve your energy levels, help control your blood sugar and reduce your risk of heart disease in addition to improving your bone health and immunity. It doesn't mean you have to be a saint every day, or turn to extreme diets, but eating more fruit and vegetables never hurt anyone. Cutting back on alcohol is a good idea – you may not realise that it is actually a class 1 carcinogen, and there is no 'safe level'. Drinking more than 14 units a week has been linked with an increased incidence of:

- Mouth cancer, throat cancer, colon and breast cancer
- Stroke
- Heart disease, palpitations, high blood pressure
- Liver disease (cirrhosis and fatty liver disease)
- Brain damage
- Damage to the nervous system

- Depression and anxiety
- Immune issues . . . to name a few.

So, cutting back on that is a no-brainer, as is giving up smoking. Respiratory diseases like Chronic Obstructive Pulmonary Disease (COPD) and lung cancer are also among the leading causes of death for women – currently ranking seventh in the US.[5]

Managing your weight is important, too. Being overweight puts extra stress on your heart and your joints, increases your risk of developing a metabolic disease like type 2 diabetes, and it also increases your risk of developing certain types of cancers like breast, colon and endometrial cancer. To put this into perspective, 23 out of every 1,000 women aged 50–59 will develop breast cancer. If you take combined MHT (that is oestrogen and a progestin) an additional four people will develop it. But if you are overweight or obese that figure jumps by an extra 24 cases taking the total from a base of 23 to 47/1000.[6]

What if I'm not perimenopausal yet – how prepared do I have to be?

If you're reading this and, like the woman at the wedding, you're worried about what 'fresh hell' the future holds for you, as both Harper and Mukherjee say, it may not be as bad as you think it's going to be. You may be one of those lucky ones who sail through unscathed and if not, you are now forewarned in a way that this generation and the ones before haven't been. And you now also know how all those silent changes to the blood, bones and brain could affect you and what you can do to keep yourself as healthy as possible for as long as possible. Try not to approach it with a catastrophic mindset – it can't be avoided (yet), so be proactive about your health and know your options.

Don't we just become invisible and disappear?

In 1991 feminist author Germaine Greer wrote a book about menopause called *The Change*. She talked about menopause, or the climacteric as she preferred to call it, in soothing terms, almost like palliative care. In fact, she called it the 'ante-chamber of death' – that's cheery. Just before we slide on into that chamber she does have a few warm(ish) words of comfort: 'Only when the stress of the climacteric is over can the aging woman realize that autumn can be long, golden, milder and warmer than summer, and is the most productive season of the year.' So, as we slowly fade away towards our final winter of discontent, she argues we're missing the big picture and should embrace 'the change'. 'It is quite impossible to explain to younger women that this new invisibility, like calm and indifference, is a desirable condition.' Much of her argument seems to centre on coming to terms with our loss of youth and beauty – finally being free of ego and using our newfound invisibility to become invincible and revel in life and all it has to offer.

And I think many of Greer's generation have indeed been revelling in all life has to offer, but very visibly. They aren't going down quietly. Look at popular culture – Helen Mirren is at the time of writing, 79. Dame Judi Dench is 90. Cher is 78, Meryl Streep is 75 – and they're still strutting their stuff on stage and screen. Gloria Steinem at 91 is still involved with feminist advocacy and publishing, as we've learnt.

And Gen X and the younger boomers don't appear to be any different. Political pickings are looking a little slim at the moment, but we have the leader of the EU Ursula von de Leyen at 66, the president of Mexico Claudia Sheinbaum is 62, and Kamala Harris is a spring chicken at 60. In finance and business we have Christine Lagarde, president of the European Central Bank, who is 69. Mary Barra, chief executive of General Motors, is 63, Jane Fraser is the first female CEO of Citibank at 57 and Mellody Hobson, author and former chair of Starbucks, is 55. Over in the tech world, 63-year-old Safra Catz is the CEO of Oracle. Recently returned from many months orbiting the earth we have the amazing astronaut, 62-year-old Suni Williams, and the acting administrator of NASA is 65-year-old Janet Petro. So, there's some inspiration!

And taboos have been broken. While psychiatrist David Reuben, who described postmenopausal women as being 'as close as she can to being a man . . . not really a man but no longer a functional woman'[7] in his 1969 book *Everything You Always Wanted to Know about Sex but Were Afraid to Ask*, nothing could be further from the truth. In 2021 *Sex and the City* tackled relationships and intimacy at midlife. I didn't love it, unfortunately. I thought it was stereotypical and a bit trite, but it was a step towards breaking down barriers by discussing the sneak attack of a 'flash period' that suddenly arrives without warning after many months of drought, and that you can still have a sex life if you want one, in spite of your reproductive status.

Twenty years earlier *Absolutely Fabulous* didn't shy away from it either. Patsy was diagnosed with osteoporosis, with record-breakingly low bone density that Edina's daughter, Saffron, said rendered her little more than 'gristle clinging on to bone powder'. Edina proffered a hormone patch as a solution which Saffron reminded her came with risks. That of course didn't worry Patsy, who proclaimed, 'How many times have I nearly overdosed? I think I can handle a patch' – that is, of course, if she could get her hands on one in today's ongoing global shortages.

Then, of course, in 2019 there was the monumental *Fleabag* soliloquy written by Phoebe Waller-Bridge, delivered by Dame Kristin Scott Thomas. Just in case you'd forgotten, she detailed the pain women go through throughout their reproductive lives and how they've almost come to terms with it when 'the f***ing menopause' strikes, which she goes on to say is 'the most wonderful f***ing thing in the world' because, despite the bladder betrayal, prolapses and hot sweats, you're finally free and 'just a person'. And as she says, that's got to be something to look forward to.

So, we're far from being an invisible generation. In fact, I sometimes wonder if we ever were, and if we do a disservice to women from past generations by thinking two things – 1) it's only youth that achieves change, and 2) that women aren't that big a part of any change that is achieved. Remember, the suffragette Emmeline Pankhurst was 69 when women over the age of 21 got the vote in the UK. Yes, she had spent 55 years or so fighting for it, but she didn't give up. We may be underrepresented but we do make a mark, and age is not a barrier. We're not done yet!

What you can do for yourself

We saw in the last chapter what you can do to help make the system better as well as adopting the many suggestions throughout the book for improving your health. But how can you advocate for yourself in a system that's still not stacked in your favour, especially when it comes to short medical consultations where you're only supposed to turn up with one symptom.

1 Come prepared – GPs are trained in a system called ICE – ideas, concerns and expectations. So tell them what your idea is, why it concerns you and what you expect – then you're speaking their language. Tell them what your symptoms are, how much and when they bother you, how long you've had them for, what effect they have on you and why you think they're related to menopause, and what outcome you are looking for.

2 Keep a record of your symptoms. This will help with the discussion and there are plenty of symptom trackers you can download, or you can find them on apps, or even a good old-fashioned pen and paper will do. Write down the symptoms and rate them in severity and frequency over time so your doctor can see what's been affecting you. Take this with you to show the doctor. There is one on the Menopause Research and Education Fund website under resources: https://mref.uk/menopause-symptom-checker/

3 Book a longer consultation if you feel you need more time to discuss your symptoms.

4 Take a friend or family member along to the consultation if you think that would help – someone to vouch for the way you feel.

5 Know the treatment options – this includes both the types of MHT that are available and the lifestyle changes that can help. Show you've done you've homework and have some idea of what you want, and that you understand the possible risks and benefits.

6 Don't be afraid to ask questions – why is this the best option for you, what are the alternatives, are there any other things we should test for/rule out or try?

7 If your doctor disagrees that your symptoms are related to menopause, don't be afraid to ask why, and perhaps suggest a trial to see whether or not MHT works for you.

8 Take in some documents that can back your argument, like some recent journal articles or a copy of current Menopause Society or NICE national guidelines may help. You can suggest that they may find these interesting and that perhaps they could take a look and you can discuss it at your next appointment? Be engaging, not confrontational – this might work better than telling them

that they clearly have no idea and are gaslighting you before you storm out the door.

9 If you still get nowhere, you can ask to see someone else at the practice who has an interest in menopause, or ask to be referred to a menopause clinic or specialist.

10 And if they still refuse, you can write a letter to the practice manager, send your supporting documents and outline why you feel they aren't operating within current evidence-based guidelines.

(By the way, if you are a doctor and are reading this, please don't take this personally because you are appreciated, but please don't have a cup on your desk that says: 'Don't confuse your Google search with my medical degree.' As amusing as that may be for you, nothing says, 'I'm not listening to you' louder than that, and your consultation has nowhere to go but downwards. If you're thinking 'surely no doctor would do that?', they do, I've seen it, and I've had it said to me. Suffice to say it didn't go down well – and as some endometriosis sufferers have stated 'please don't confuse your medical degree with my lifetime of pain'. No one wins here – so best to be avoided. It may be best to just take the cup home.)

Ultimately the decisions you make about how to handle your menopause are yours and involve shared care and informed consent between you and your doctor/s. You are an active participant in this. If you do decide on MHT, bear in mind it can be a case of trial and error once you start. You may not get on with it well, there could be symptoms or side effects that take time to settle, and you may have to chop and change varieties and doses until you find what suits you. And just when you thought you had it all sorted you may find this needs to change as your symptoms change.

But you are now in a great place. It may not be perfect, but you have so much information at your fingertips and we aren't done yet in changing the system. As much as I hate these marketing terms – 'baby boomers' and 'gen X' – we have beaten a drum that has changed the face of menopause and turned a 'moment' into a movement. As they say, the revolution may not be televised but the push for change will continue to ensure the gaps in gender health spans and data are closed along with the economic disparities created by simply being born with ovaries.

Many of us will live a good 30–50 years, maybe even more, after menopause, so looking after our health now and every day from now on is so important. To do that we need to make sure we have the evidence-based information and all the options, medical, non-medical and lifestyle-wise, available to us so we can spend that time in good health and maintain our independence. These will be challenges in an ageing population with limited resources, because it has to be backed by funded policy, and we will only achieve that if we have unified voices across the board.

Remember though, this is about you. It is your menopause, your health, your future, your choices. You do it your way – because, in the end it's absolutely no one else's business – and, you really are worth it!

Notes

Preface

1 The global population of postmenopausal women is growing. In 2021, women aged 50 and over accounted for 26 per cent of all women and girls globally. This was up from 22 per cent 10 years earlier. Additionally, women are living longer. Globally, a woman aged 60 years in 2019 could expect to live on average another 21 years.

2 (2024) Funding research on women's health. *Nat Rev Bioeng*, 2, 797–98. doi: 10.1038/s44222-024-00253-7

3 https://nihr.opendatasoft.com/pages/nihr-awards-filters/-value-of-awards#-value-of-awards

Chapter 1

1 Jermyn, D. (2024) Whose menopause revolution? Investigating the UK's 'Davina effect' and the contemporary menopause market. *European Journal of Cultural Studies*, 0(0). doi: 10.1177/13675494241287931

2 Hansard. https://hansard.parliament.uk/commons/2022-06-09/debates/5EEB4A70-CDA6-4474-B440-3CF855FD4713/Menopause

3 https://www.health.gov.au/sites/default/files/2025-02/government-response-to-inquiry-issues-related-to-menopause-and-perimenopause.pdf

4 https://www.nytimes.com/2023/07/28/podcasts/the-daily/menopause-symptoms-treatment.html

5 https://www.newsweek.com/why-lauren-hutton-smiling-hormones-158001

6 https://thebms.org.uk/2022/05/bms-comment-on-channel-4-programme-davina-mccall-sex-myths-and-the-menopause/

7 https://thebms.org.uk/publications/consensus-statements/primary-prevention-of-coronary-heart-disease-in-women/

8 https://thebms.org.uk/2024/07/bms-statement-on-testosterone-2/

9 https://thebms.org.uk/2024/11/british-menopause-society-statement-on-hrt-dosages/

10 Panay, N., Ang, S.B., Cheshire, R., Goldstein, S.R., Maki, P. and Nappi, R.E. On behalf of the International Menopause Society Board (2024) Menopause and MHT in 2024: Addressing the key controversies – an International Menopause Society White Paper. *Climacteric*. doi: 10.1080/13697137.2024.2394950

11 https://thebms.org.uk/about-the-charity/our-people/#:~:text=To%20date%2C%20Sara%20has%20served,1%20million%20and%20 2%2C500%20members

233

12   https://www.statista.com/statistics/1488562/number-of-us-active-
      primary-care-physicians-by-field/#:~:text=As%20of%20May%20
      2024%2C%20there,the%20field%20of%20internal%20medicine

13   https://www.bls.gov/oes/2023/may/oes291215.htm

14   https://www.ibisworld.com/united-states/industry/gynecologists-
      obstetricians/6008/

15   (2024) Time for a balanced conversation about menopause. *The Lancet*,
      403(10430), 877.

16   Samarasekera, U. (2024) Martha Hickey: Responding to the complexity
      of menopause. *The Lancet*, 403(10430), 893.

17   (2024) Time for a balanced conversation about menopause, *The Lancet*,
      403(10430), 877.

18   Hickey, M. et al. (2024) An empowerment model for managing
      menopause. *The Lancet*, 403(10430), 947–957.

19   https://msmagazine.com/2024/04/15/menopause-treatment-the-lancet/

20   https://menopause.org/wp-content/uploads/professional/2023-
      nonhormone-therapy-position-statement.pdf

21   https://www.nice.org.uk/guidance/ng23/chapter/recommendations#
      managing-symptoms-associated-with-menopause-in-people-aged-40-or-over

22   Sibbald, B. (2002) US estrogen plus progestin HRT trial stopped due to
      increased risk of breast cancer, stroke and heart attack. *CMAJ*, 6 August,
      167(3), 294. PMCID: PMC117494.

23   Rossouw, J.E., Anderson, G.L., Prentice, R.L., LaCroix, A.Z., Kooperberg,
      C., Stefanick, M.L., Jackson, R.D., Beresford, S.A., Howard, B.V.,
      Johnson, K.C., Kotchen, J.M. and Ockene, J. (2002) Writing group
      for the Women's Health Initiative Investigators. Risks and benefits of
      estrogen plus progestin in healthy postmenopausal women: Principal
      results. From the Women's Health Initiative randomized controlled
      trial. *JAMA*, 17 July, 288(3), 321–33. doi: 10.1001/jama.288.3.321.
      PMID: 12117397.

24   https://thebms.org.uk/wp-content/uploads/2023/01/WHC-Infographics-
      JANUARY-2023-BreastCancerRisks.pdf

25   Stute, P., Marsden, J., Salih, N. and Cagnacci, A. (2023) Reappraising
      21 years of the WHI study: Putting the findings in context for clinical
      practice. *Maturitas*, 174, 8–13, doi: 10.1016/j.maturitas.2023.04.271

26   Clark, J.H. (2006) A critique of Women's Health Initiative Studies
      (2002–2006). *Nucl Recept Signal*, 30 October, 4, e023. doi: 10.1621/
      nrs.04023. PMID: 17088939; PMCID: PMC1630688.

27   Townsend, J. (1998) Hormone replacement therapy: Assessment of
      present use, costs, and trends. *British Journal of General Practice*. https://
      bjgp.org/content/48/427/955.short

28   Menon, U., Burnell, M., Sharma, A., Gentry-Maharaj, A., Fraser, L., Ryan, A., Parmar, M., Hunter, M. and Jacobs, I. (2007) UKCTOCS Group: Decline in use of hormone therapy among postmenopausal women in the United Kingdom. *Menopause*, 14, 462–67. doi: 10.1097/01.gme.0000243569.70946.9d

29   Cagnacci, A. and Venier, M. (2019) The controversial history of hormone replacement therapy. *Medicina* (Kaunas), 18 September, 55(9), 602. doi: 10.3390/medicina55090602. PMID: 31540401; PMCID: PMC6780820.

30   https://www.gov.uk/government/news/hundreds-of-thousands-of-women-experiencing-menopause-symptoms-to-get-cheaper-hormone-replacement-therapy

31   Anderer, S. (2024) Only about 5% of US women now use menopausal hormone therapy. *JAMA*, 332(21), 1779. doi:10.1001/jama.2024.22564

32   Avis, N.E., Crawford, S.L. and Green, R. (2018) Vasomotor symptoms across the menopause transition: Differences among women. *Obstet Gynecol Clin North Am*, December, 45(4), 629–40. doi: 10.1016/j.ogc.2018.07.005. Epub 25 October 2018. PMID: 30401547; PMCID: PMC6226273.

33   https://www.menopause.org.au/hp/gp-hp-resources/lancet-series-on-menopause-2024

Chapter 2

1   https://www.aarp.org/health/drugs-supplements/testosterone-for-women.html#:~:text=Despite%20the%20hype%2C%20the%20only,or%20difficulties%20in%20your%20relationship

2   https://drstreicher.substack.com/p/is-your-doctor-really-a-menopause

3   https://www.gov.uk/government/publications/womens-health-strategy-for-england/womens-health-strategy-for-england#menopause

4   https://www.youtube.com/watch?v=J3VuNBw3Nb8

5   https://menopausesupport.co.uk/wp-content/uploads/2021/05/Web-info-Shocking-Disparity-in-Menopause-Training-in-Medical-Schools-1.pdf

6   Kling, J.M. et al. (2019) Menopause management knowledge in postgraduate family medicine, internal medicine, and obstetrics and gynecology residents: A cross-sectional survey. *Mayo Clinic Proceedings*, 94(2), 242–53. https://www.mayoclinicproceedings.org/article/S0025-6196(18)30701-8/abstract

7   Allen, J.T. et al. (2023) Needs assessment of menopause education in United States obstetrics and gynecology residency training programs. *Menopause*, October 1, 30(10): 1002-1005. doi: 10.1097/GME.0000000000002234. Epub 2023 Aug 8. PMID: 37738034. https://pubmed.ncbi.nlm.nih.gov/37738034/

8   Barber, K. and Charles, A. (2023) Barriers to accessing effective treatment and support for menopausal symptoms: A qualitative study capturing the behaviours, beliefs and experiences of key stakeholders. *Patient Prefer Adherence*, 15 November, 17, 2971–80. doi: 10.2147/PPA. S430203. PMID: 38027078; PMCID: PMC10657761

9   https://www.mumsnet.com/articles/gps-and-menopause-survey

10 It is not within the remit of central government to require that one member of clinical staff in every GP surgery has training on menopause. As set out above, menopause care is a core competency of all qualified GPs.

11 https://www.judiciary.uk/prevention-of-future-death-reports/jacqueline-anne-potter-prevention-of-future-deaths-report/

12 Government response to inquiry – Issues related to menopause and perimenopause, Recommendation 12. https://www.health.gov.au/resources/publications/government-response-to-inquiry-issues-related-to-menopause-and-perimenopause?language=en

13 https://thebms.org.uk/wp-content/uploads/2023/04/14-BMS-TfC-Progestogens-and-endometrial-protection-APR2023-A.pdf

Chapter 3

1   Avis, N.E., Crawford, S.L., Greendale, G. et al. (2015) Duration of menopausal vasomotor symptoms over the menopause transition. *JAMA Intern Med*, 175(4), 531–39. doi: 10.1001/jamainternmed.2014.8063

2   https://thebms.org.uk/wp-content/uploads/2024/04/05-BMS-ConsensusStatement-Premature-ovarian-insufficiency-POI-APRIL2024-C.pdf

3   Li, M., Zhu, Y., Wei, J., Chen, L., Chen, S. and Lai, D. (2022) The global prevalence of premature ovarian insufficiency: A systematic review and meta-analysis. *Climacteric*, April 26(2), 95–102. doi: 10.1080/13697137.2022.2153033. Epub 15 December 2022. PMID: 36519275.

4   https://cks.nice.org.uk/topics/menopause/diagnosis/diagnosis-of-menopause-perimenopause/

5   https://www.nice.org.uk/guidance/ng23/chapter/Recommendations#diagnosing-and-managing-premature-ovarian-insufficiency-in-people-under-40

6   ESHRE, ASRM, CREWHIRL and IMS Guideline Group on POI; Panay, N., Anderson, R.A., Bennie, A., Cedars, M., Davies, M., Ee, C., Gravholt, C.H., Kalantaridou, S., Kallen, A., Kim, K.Q., Misrahi, M., Mousa, A., Nappi, R.E., Rocca, W.A., Ruan, X., Teede, H., Vermeulen, N., Vogt, E. and Vincent, A.J. (2024) Evidence-based guideline: Premature ovarian insufficiency.

Climacteric, December, 27(6), 510–20. doi: 10.1080/13697137.2024. 2423213. Epub 8 December 2024. PMID: 39647506.

7   https://www.australianpharmacist.com.au/cup-of-tea-bex-good-lie-down/

8   https://www.historyhit.com/mothers-little-helper-the-history-of-valium/

9   https://pmc.ncbi.nlm.nih.gov/articles/PMC2424120/#b40

10 Dean-Jones, L. (1994) *Women in the Classical World: Image and Text.* New York and London: Oxford University Press. p. 199.

11 https://www.rcn.org.uk/library-exhibitions/Womens-health-wandering-womb#:~:text=Women%20have%20long%20been%20seen,sex%2C%20both%20physically%20and%20mentally

12 https://collection.sciencemuseumgroup.org.uk/objects/co91167/vaginal-speculum-for-applying-leeches

13 https://www.theatlantic.com/magazine/archive/2019/10/the-secret-power-of-menopause/596662/

14 https://www.urmc.rochester.edu/ob-gyn/ur-medicine-menopause-and-womens-health/menopause-blog/february-2016/the-history-of-estrogen

15 https://www.nytimes.com/2002/07/10/us/hormone-replacement-study-a-shock-to-the-medical-system.html

16 https://www.ucpress.edu/books/encounters-with-aging/paper

17 Brown, D.E., Sievert, L.L., Morrison, L.A., Reza, A.M. and Mills, P.S. (2009) Do Japanese American women really have fewer hot flashes than European Americans? The Hilo Women's Health Study. *Menopause*, Sept–Oct, 16(5), 870–76. doi: 10.1097/gme.0b013e31819d88da. PMID: 19367185; PMCID: PMC2746710.

18 Li, J., Luo, M., Tang, R., Sun, X., Wang, Y., Liu, B., Cui, J., Liu, G., Lin, S. and Chen, R. (2020) Vasomotor symptoms in aging Chinese women: Findings from a prospective cohort study. *Climacteric*, February, 23(1), 46–52. doi: 10.1080/13697137.2019.1628734. Epub 4 July 2019. PMID: 31269826.

19 Wang, X., Wang, L., Di, J., Zhang, X. and Zhao, G. (2021) Prevalence and risk factors for menopausal symptoms in middle-aged Chinese women: A community-based cross-sectional study. *Menopause*, 30 August, 28(11), 1271–78. doi: 10.1097/GME.0000000000001850. PMID: 34469934; PMCID: PMC8547757.

20 Im, E.O., Seung, H.L. and Chee, W. (2010) Subethnic differences in the menopausal symptom experience of Asian American midlife women. *J Transcult Nurs*, April, 21(2), 123–33. doi: 10.1177/1043659609357639. PMID: 20220032; PMCID: PMC2838208.

21 Yu, Q., Chae, H.D., Hsiao, S.-M., Xie, J., Blogg, M., Sumarsono, B. and Kim, S. (2022) Prevalence, severity, and associated factors in women in East Asia with moderate-to-severe vasomotor symptoms associated with menopause. *Menopause*, May. doi: 10.1097/GME.0000000000001949

22 Walker, M.D., Liu, X.S., Stein, E., Zhou, B., Bezati, E., McMahon, D.J., Udesky, J., Liu, G., Shane, E., Guo, X.E. and Bilezikian, J.P. (2011) Differences in bone microarchitecture between postmenopausal Chinese-American and white women. *J Bone Miner Res*, July, 26(7), 1392–98. doi: 10.1002/jbmr.352. PMID: 21305606; PMCID: PMC3558983.

23 Zhang, Y., Wang, J., Zu, Y. and Hu, Q. (2021) Attitudes of Chinese college students toward aging and living independently in the context of china's modernization: A qualitative study. *Front Psychol*, 31 May, 12, 609736. doi: 10.3389/fpsyg.2021.609736. PMID: 34135797; PMCID: PMC8200472.

24 https://content.csbs.utah.edu/~hawkes/Hawkes_al89hardworking HadzaGrams.pdf

25 https://www.smithsonianmag.com/science-nature/how-much-did-grandmothers-influence-human-evolution-180976665/

26 Hooper, P.L., Gurvern, M., Winking, J. and Hillard, S.K. (2015) Inclusive fitness and differential productivity across the life course determine intergenerational transfers in a small-scale human society. *Proceedings*, 282(1803) doi: 10.1098/rspb.2014.2808

27 Engelhardt, S.C, Bergeron, P., Gagnon, A., Dillon, l. and Pelletier, F. (2019) Using geographical distance as a potential proxy for help in the assessment of the grandmother hypothesis. *Curr Biol*, 29, 651–656, e3.

28 Madrigal, L. and Meléndez-Obando, M. (2008) Grandmothers' longevity negatively affects daughters' fertility. *The American Journal of Phyicla Anthropology*, June, 136(2), 223–9. doi: 10.1002/ajpa.20798. https://pubmed.ncbi.nlm.nih.gov/18322917/

29 Roser, M. (2020) It's not just about child mortality, life expectancy increased at all ages. https://ourworldindata.org/its-not-just-about-child-mortality-life-expectancy-improved-at-all-ages

30 Amundsen, D.W. and Diers, D.J. (1970) The age of menopause in classical Greece and Rome. *Human Biology*, 42(1), 79–86. http://www.jstor.org/stable/41449006

Chapter 4

1 Rutter, J. (1808) A case of Hysteraglia. *Edinb Med Surg J*, April, 4(14), 168–177. https://pubmed.ncbi.nlm.nih.gov/30331289/

2 https://committees.parliament.uk/publications/45909/documents/228040/default/

3 Manchanda, R., Gaba, F., Talaulikar, V., Pundir, J., Gessler, S., Davies, M., and Menon, U. (2022) Risk-reducing salpingo-oophorectomy and the use of hormone replacement therapy below the age of natural menopause. Scientific Impact Paper No. 66, *BJOG*. January, 129(1): e16–e34, Royal College of Obstetricians and Gynaecologists. doi: 10.1111/1471-0528.16896. Epub 2021 Oct 20. PMID: 34672090; PMCID: PMC7614764.

4 https://www.nhs.uk/conditions/hysteroscopy/

5 Rowlands, S., Oloto, E. and Horwell, D.H. (2016) Intrauterine devices and risk of uterine perforation: Current perspectives. *Open Access Journal of Contraception*, 7, 19–32. doi: 10.2147/OAJC.S85546

6 https://www.hysteroscopyaction.org.uk/caph-survey-results/

7 https://pmc.ncbi.nlm.nih.gov/articles/PMC8212159/#:~:text=There%20were%2071%2C000%20hysteroscopies%20performed,which%20almost%20half%20were%20therapeutic

8 https://researchbriefings.files.parliament.uk/documents/CDP-2023-0024/CDP-2023-0024.pdf

9 https://www.england.nhs.uk/2023/11/women-urged-to-take-up-nhs-cervical-screening-invitations/

10 https://www.gov.uk/government/publications/health-matters-making-cervical-screening-more-accessible/health-matters-making-cervical-screening-more-accessible--2

11 https://committees.parliament.uk/publications/45909/documents/228040/default/

12 https://www.gov.uk/government/publications/womens-health-strategy-for-england/womens-health-strategy-for-england#menopause

13 https://www.fawcettsociety.org.uk/Handlers/Download.ashx?IDMF=ab18c943-9c75-4320-8bb4-ae781d2dedec

14 https://mcusercontent.com/09f8a3d6ac97af32198dc2c74/files/4945540e-9c8b-2840-19f1-028d89546a34/APPG_Menopause_Inquiry_Concluding_Report_12.10.22.pdf

15 https://www.gov.uk/government/calls-for-evidence/womens-health-strategy-call-for-evidence/outcome/3fa4a313-f7a5-429a-b68d-0eb0be15e696#womens-voices-1

16 Ibid.

17 https://www.mumsnet.com/articles/gps-and-menopause-survey

18 Barber, K. and Charles, A. (2023) Barriers to accessing effective treatment and support for menopausal symptoms: A qualitative study capturing the behaviours, beliefs and experiences of key stakeholders. *Patient Prefer Adherence*, 15 November, 17, 2971–80. doi: 10.2147/PPA.S430203. PMID: 38027078; PMCID: PMC10657761.

19 https://swhr.org/health_focus_area/menopause/

20 https://www.engage.england.nhs.uk/safety-and-innovation/menopause-in-the-workplace/

21 Hill, K. (1996) The demography of menopause. *Maturitas*, 23(2), 113–27. ISSN 0378-5122. doi: 10.1016/0378-5122(95)00968-X. https://www.sciencedirect.com/science/article/pii/037851229500968X

Chapter 5

1   https://www.mckinsey.com/mhi/our-insights/closing-the-womens-health-gap-a-1-trillion-dollar-opportunity-to-improve-lives-and-economies

2   https://www.actuarialpost.co.uk/article/mums-with-children-and-work-part-time-lose-pension-savings-18818.htm

3   https://member.railwayspensions.co.uk/knowledge-hub/news-and-views/blog/rps-blog/2024/03/06/mind-the-gender-pension-gap

4   https://www.nowpensions.com/app/uploads/2024/02/gender-pensions-gap-report-24.pdf

5   https://www.kingsfund.org.uk/insight-and-analysis/data-and-charts/key-facts-figures-adult-social-care

6   https://www.carersuk.org/policy-and-research/key-facts-and-figures/#:~:text=Our Facts about carers document

7   https://www.carersuk.org/reports/valuing-carers/

8   https://www.carersuk.org/policy-and-research/key-facts-and-figures/#:~:text=Our Facts about carers document

9   https://ifs.org.uk/sites/default/files/2025-03/WP202510-The-menopause-penalty_0.pdf

10 Faubion, S.S. et al. (2023) Impact of menopause symptoms on women in the workplace. https://www.mayoclinicproceedings.org/pb-assets/Health%20Advance/journals/jmcp/JMCP4097_proof.pdf

11 https://www.bupa.com/news-and-press/press-releases/2021/bupa-launches-menopause-helpline

12 https://magnificentmidlife.com/blog/is-it-true-900000-women-left-work-because-of-menopause/

13 https://www.fawcettsociety.org.uk/Handlers/Download.ashx?IDMF=9672cf45-5f13-4b69-8882-1e5e643ac8a6

14 https://www.bma.org.uk/media/2913/bma-challenging-the-culture-on-menopause-for-working-doctors-report-aug-2020.pdf

15 https://www.cipd.org/uk/knowledge/reports/menopause-workplace-experiences/#:~:text=Employers%20are%20losing%20around%20one,further%206%25%20have%20left%20work

16 https://www.simplyhealth.co.uk/news-and-articles/35-million-women-have-considered-quitting-job-due-to-menopause-and-menstrual-health-symptoms

17 https://www.nhsconfed.org/publications/womens-health-economics#:~:text=Employing%20the%20methodology%20that%20was,due%20to%20severe%20perimenopause%20and

18 https://committees.parliament.uk/writtenevidence/39340/html/

19   https://www.gov.uk/government/publications/health-matters-preventing-
      cardiovascular-disease/health-matters-preventing-cardiovascular-disease#:
      ~:text=Yearly%20healthcare%20costs%20in%20England,economy%20
      of%20%C2%A315.8%20billion

20   https://hsrc.himmelfarb.gwu.edu/cgi/viewcontent.cgi?article=1269
      &context=sphhs_policy_facpubs

21   https://www.healthdata.org/research-analysis/gbd

22   Daly, C.A., Clemens, F., Sendon, J.L. et al. (2005) The clinical characteristics
      and investigations planned in patients with stable angina presenting to
      cardiologists in Europe: From the Euro Heart Survey of Stable Angina.
      Eur Heart J, 26, 996–1010.

23   https://www.ahajournals.org/doi/10.1161/jaha.116.004972

24   https://www.thelancet.com/journals/eclinm/article/PIIS2589-5370(19)
      30183-X/fulltext#:~:text=Interpretation,fatal%20ADRs%20among%20
      male%20reports

25   Radmaker, M. (2001) Do women have more adverse drug reactions? *Am
      J Clin Dermatol*, 2(6), 349–51, doi: 10.2165/00128071-200102060-00001

26   https://news.harvard.edu/gazette/story/2023/12/women-more-likely-to-
      suffer-drug-side-effects-but-reason-may-not-be-biology/

27   https://www.immdsreview.org.uk/downloads/IMMDSReview_Web.pdf

28   https://www.sciencemuseum.org.uk/objects-and-stories/medicine/
      thalidomide

29   http://news.bbc.co.uk/1/hi/8428838.stm

30   https://www.abc.net.au/news/2014-02-07/supreme-court-formally-
      approves-2489m-class-action-for-thalido/5245034

31   https://orwh.od.nih.gov/toolkit/recruitment/history#3

32   https://www.ncbi.nlm.nih.gov/books/NBK236531/?report=reader

33   https://www.nih.gov/about-nih/what-we-do/budget#:~:text=The%20
      NIH%20invests%20most%20of,research%20for%20the%20
      American%20people

34   https://www.nihr.ac.uk/news/nihr-spends-ps13bn-delivering-world-
      leading-research-shows-2022-23-annual-report#:~:text=Financial%20
      report,%2C%20was%20%C2%

35   https://data.worldbank.org/indicator/NY.GDP.MKTP.CD?locations=GB

36   Steinberg, J.R., Turner, B.E., Weeks, B.T., Magnani, C.J., Wong, B.O.,
      Rodriguez, F., Yee, L.M. and Cullen, M.R. (2021) Analysis of female
      enrollment and participant sex by burden of disease in US clinical trials
      between 2000 and 2020. *JAMA Netw Open*, 1 June, 1, 4(6), e2113749.
      doi: 10.1001/jamanetworkopen.2021.13749. PMID: 34143192; PMCID:
      PMC8214160.

37 Sosinsky, A.Z. et al. (2022) Enrollment of female participants in United States drug and device phase 1–3 clinical trials between 2016 and 2019. *Contemporary Clinical Trials*, April, 115, 106718. doi: 10.1016/j. cct.2022.106718

38 Bierer, B.E., Meloney, L.G., Ahmed, H.R. and White, S.A. (2022) Advancing the inclusion of underrepresented women in clinical research. *Cell Rep Med*, 7 Mar, 3(4), 100553. doi: 10.1016/j.xcrm.2022. 100553. PMID: 35492242; PMCID: PMC9043984. https://pmc.ncbi. nlm.nih.gov/articles/PMC9043984/#abs0010

39 https://time.com/7171341/gender-gap-medical-research/

40 https://www.nihr.ac.uk/blog/improving-research-through-inclusive-design-sex-and-gender

41 https://www.cdc.gov/tuskegee/about/index.html

42 https://www.nytimes.com/1972/07/26/archives/syphilis-victims-in-us-study-went-untreated-for-40-years-syphilis.html

43 https://pubmed.ncbi.nlm.nih.gov/17226823/#:~:text=Enslaved%20 and%20free%20African%20Americans,medical%20schools%20for%20 anatomic%20dissection

44 https://www.smithsonianmag.com/smart-news/mothers-of-gynecology-monument-honors-enslaved-women-180980064/

45 Reflection on Black and Ethnic Minority Participation in Clinical Trials.

46 https://www.bbc.co.uk/news/55747544

47 https://www.bbc.co.uk/news/uk-england-bristol-55937548

48 https://static.project2025.org/2025_MandateForLeadership_FULL.pdf

49 https://www.nhsconfed.org/publications/womens-health-economics

50 https://www.gov.uk/government/publications/womens-health-strategy-for-england/womens-health-strategy-for-england#menopause

Chapter 6

1 https://www.forbes.com/sites/njgoldston/2018/08/21/how-to-harness-the-untapped-spending-power-of-the-50-ish-super-consumer/ #2759954616db

2 https://www.globenewswire.com/news-release/2024/11/21/2985347/0/ en/Menopause-Market-Size-to-Hit-USD-27-63-Billion-by-2033-Straits-Research.html

3 https://www.mckinsey.com/industries/consumer-packaged-goods/ our-insights/the-trends-defining-the-1-point-8-trillion-dollar-global-wellness-market-in-2024

4 https://uk.happymammoth.com/pages/hormonal-weight-assist

5 Randle, M., Mintzes, B., McCarthy, S., Pitt, H. and Thomas, S. (2024) Conflicts of interest in submissions and testimonies to an Australian

parliamentary inquiry on menopause. *Health Promotion International*, December, 39(6), daae150, doi: 10.1093/heapro/daae150

6 https://www.independent.co.uk/business/menopausal-women-spending-average-ps1-800-a-year-to-combat-symptoms-b2708072.html

7 https://cks.nice.org.uk/topics/anaemia-iron-deficiency/diagnosis/investigations/

8 Kopecky, S.L., Bauer, D.C., Gulati, M., Nieves, J.W., Singer, A.J., Toth, P.P., Underberg, J.A., Wallace, T.C. and Weaver, C.M. (2016) Lack of evidence linking calcium with or without vitamin d supplementation to cardiovascular disease in generally healthy adults: A clinical guideline from the National Osteoporosis Foundation and the American Society for Preventive Cardiology. *Ann Intern Med*, 20 December, 165(12), 867–68. doi: 10.7326/M16-1743. Epub 25 October 2016. PMID: 27776362. https://pubmed.ncbi.nlm.nih.gov/27776362/

9 https://www.nhs.uk/conditions/vitamins-and-minerals/calcium/

10 https://my.clevelandclinic.org/health/diseases/14597-hypercalcemia

11 Vyas, C.M., Manson, J.E., Sesso, H.D., Cook, N.R., Rist, P.M., Weinberg, A., Moorthy, M.V., Baker, L.D., Espeland, M.A., Yeung, L.K., Brickman, A.M. and Okereke, O.I. (2024) Effect of multivitamin-mineral supplementation versus placebo on cognitive function: Results from the clinic subcohort of the COcoa Supplement and Multivitamin Outcomes Study (COSMOS) randomized clinical trial and meta-analysis of 3 cognitive studies within COSMOS. *Am J Clin Nutr*, March, 119(3), 692–701. doi: 10.1016/j.ajcnut.2023.12.011. Epub 2024 Jan 18. PMID: 38244989; PMCID: PMC11103094. https://pubmed.ncbi.nlm.nih.gov/38244989/

12 Barnard, N.D., Kahleova, H. and Becker, R. (2024) The limited value of multivitamin supplements. *JAMA Netw Open*, 7(6), e2418965. doi:10.1001/jamanetworkopen.2024.18965

13 https://www.gao.gov/assets/gao-19-23r.pdf

14 (2015) Emergency department visits for adverse events related to dietary supplements. *N Engl J Med*, 373(16), 1531–40, doi: 10.1056/NEJMsa1504267

15 https://pharmaceutical-journal.com/article/news/drug-interactions-with-dietary-or-herbal-supplements-could-be-cause-of-hospital-stays

16 https://ods.od.nih.gov/factsheets/WYNTK-Consumer/#h2

17 https://www.food.gov.uk/business-guidance/food-supplements#legal-requirements

18 https://menopause.org/wp-content/uploads/professional/2023-nonhormone-therapy-position-statement.pdf

19 Bettany, S. (2023) The 'pinkification' of menopause: The silences and omissions of the menopause market gold-rush, Consumer Culture Theory Conference, Lund, Sweden

20   Yoon, H.S., Lee, S.R. and Chung, J.H. (2014) Long-term topical oestrogen treatment of sun-exposed facial skin in post-menopausal women does not improve facial wrinkles or skin elasticity, but induces matrix metalloproteinase-1 expression. *Acta Derm Venereol*, January, 94(1), 4–8. doi: 10.2340/00015555-1614. PMID: 23722352.

21   https://assets.ctfassets.net/md0kv0ejg0xf/4gaULAkbHbgNZtNMOgg1PI/ 91329de08abacf438fb83d99e756ee99/Alloy_M4_Report_063024.pdf

22   https://www.fda.gov/drugs/human-drug-compounding/national-academies-science-engineering-and-medicine-nasem-study-clinical-utility-treating-patients

23   Li, F.G., Fuchs, T., Deans, R., McCormack, L., Nesbitt-Hawes, E., Abbott, J. and Farnsworth, A. (2023) Vaginal epithelial histology before and after fractional CO2 laser in postmenopausal women: a double-blind, sham-controlled randomized trial. *Am J Obstet Gynecol*, September, 229(3), 278, e1–278. e9. doi: 10.1016/j.ajog.2023.05.005. Epub 14 May 2023. PMID: 37192705.

24   Phillips, C., Hillard, T., Salvatore, S., Toozs-Hobson, P. and Cardozo, L. (2020) Lasers in gynaecology. *Eur J Obstet Gynecol Reprod Biol*, August, 251, 146–55. doi: 10.1016/j.ejogrb.2020.03.034. Epub 2020 May 19. PMID: 32505055.

25   Anuradha J., Mysore, V., and Mysore, J.V. (2022) Cosmetic gynecology—An emerging field for the dermatologist. *Cosmet Dermatol*, January, 22(1), 11–118. doi: 10.1111/jocd.15484. https://pubmed.ncbi.nlm.nih.gov/ 36335587/

26   Photiou, L., Lin, M.J., Dubin, D.P., Lenskaya, V. and Khorasani, H. (2019) Review of non-invasive vulvovaginal rejuvenation. *J Eur Acad Dermatol Venereol*, April, 34(4), 716–26. doi: 10.1111/jdv.16066. Epub 5 December 2019. PMID: 31714632.

27   https://www.tga.gov.au/how-we-regulate/supply-therapeutic-good/ supply-medical-device/medical-device-post-market-reviews/post-market-review-energy-based-devices-used-vaginal-rejuvenation#information-for-consumers-and-healthcare-professionals

28   https://www.aliexpress.com/w/wholesale-menopause-vaginal-tightening-device-laser.html?spm=a2g0o.productlist.search.0

29   https://www.fda.gov/news-events/press-announcements/statement-fda-commissioner-scott-gottlieb-md-efforts-safeguard-womens-health-deceptive-health-claims

30   https://www.gov.uk/guidance/medical-devices-conformity-assessment-and-the-ukca-mark

31   https://pard.mhra.gov.uk/manufacturer-details/43332

32   https://www.ebay.co.uk/sch/i.html?_nkw=vaginal+laser&_sacat=0&_from=R40&_trksid=p2510209.m570.l1313#item5e752a229d

33 https://www.taylorwessing.com/en/insights-and-events/insights/2024/ 06/femtech-und-datenschutz

34 https://www.ncl.ac.uk/press/articles/latest/2024/03/femtech/

35 https://www.ftc.gov/news-events/news/press-releases/2021/06/ftc- finalizes-order-flo-health-fertility-tracking-app-shared-sensitive-health- data-facebook-google

36 https://www.reuters.com/legal/litigation/fertility-app-maker-flo-health- faces-consolidated-privacy-lawsuit-2021-09-03/

37 https://flo.health/newsroom/flo-response-ftc-settlement-update

38 https://orchahealth.com/period-tracker-apps-share-data/

39 Hamper, J. (2024) Babies are a massive money spinner': Data, reproductive labour and the commodification of pre-motherhood in fertility and pregnancy apps. *New Media & Society*, 0(0). doi: 10.1177/14614448241262805

40 https://www.femtechworld.co.uk/features/compliance-is-a-journey- how-femtech-companies-could-navigate-privacy-and-clinical-safety- requirements/

41 https://www.mckinsey.com/mhi/our-insights/closing-the-womens- health-gap-a-1-trillion-dollar-opportunity-to-improve-lives-and- economies

42 https://whamnow.org/wp-content/uploads/2025/01/WHAM-report- 011525.pdf

Chapter 7

1 Conde, D.M., Verdade, R.C., Valadares, A.L.R., Mella, L.F.B., Pedro, A.O. and Costa-Paiva, L. (2021) Menopause and cognitive impairment: A narrative review of current knowledge. *World J Psychiatry*, 19 August, 11(8), 412–28. doi: 10.5498/wjp.v11.i8.412. PMID: 34513605; PMCID: PMC8394691.

2 https://www.letstalkmenopause.org/podcast-episodes/menopause-and- the-female-brain

3 Mosconi, L., Berti, V., Dyke, J., Schelbaum, E., Jett, S., Loughlin, L., Jang, G., Rahman, A., Hristov, H., Pahlajani, S., Andrews, R., Matthews, D., Etingin, O., Ganzer, C., de Leon, M., Isaacson, R. and Brinton, R.D. (2021) Menopause impacts human brain structure, connectivity, energy metabolism, and amyloid-beta deposition. *Sci Rep*, 9 June, 11(1), 10867. doi: 10.1038/s41598-021-90084-y. PMID: 34108509; PMCID: PMC8190071.

4 https://www.letstalkmenopause.org/podcast-episodes/menopause-and- the-female-brain

5   Sperling, R.A., Karlawish, J. and Johnson, K.A. (2013) Preclinical
    Alzheimer disease – the challenges ahead. *Nat Rev Neurol*, 9, 54–58. doi:
    10.1038/nrneurol.2012.241

6   https://jamanetwork.com/journals/jamainternalmedicine/article-abstract/
    2665382

7   (2023) Systematic review and meta-analysis of the effects of menopause
    hormone therapy on risk of Alzheimer's disease and dementia. *Aging
    Neurosci*, 23 October, 15. doi: 10.3389/fnagi.2023.1260427

8   Kim, Y.J., Soto, M., Branigan, G.L., Rodgers, K. and Brinton, R.D.
    (2021) Association between menopausal hormone therapy and risk
    of neurodegenerative diseases: Implications for precision hormone
    therapy. *Alzheimer's & Dementia*, 13 May, 7(1), e12174. doi: 10.1002/
    trc2.12174. PMID: 34027024; PMCID: PMC8118114.

9   https://edition.cnn.com/2023/11/02/health/hormone-replacement-
    dementia-wellness/index.html

10 Mosconi, L., Nerattini, M., Matthews, D.C. et al. (2024) In vivo brain
    estrogen receptor density by neuroendocrine aging and relationships
    with cognition and symptomatology. *Sci Rep*, 14, 12680. doi: 10.1038/
    s41598-024-62820-7

11 https://news.weill.cornell.edu/news/2024/06/scans-show-brains-
    estrogen-activity-changes-during-menopause#:~:text=Credit%3A%20
    Mosconi%20lab.,researchers%20at%20Weill%20Cornell%20Medicine

12 Bove, R., Secor, E., Chibnik, L.B., Barnes, L.L., Schneider, J.A., Bennett,
    D.A. and De Jager, P.L. (2024) Age at surgical menopause influences
    cognitive decline and Alzheimer pathology in older women. *Neurology*,
    21 January, 82(3), 222–29. doi: 10.1212/WNL.0000000000000033. Epub
    11 December 2013. PMID: 24336141; PMCID: PMC3902759.

13 https://www.oprahdaily.com/life/health/a45599227/hormone-
    replacement-alzheimers-risk/

14 https://www.express.co.uk/life-style/health/1920982/expert-dementia-
    prevention-women-menopause

15 https://www.sciencedaily.com/releases/2021/07/210712092238.htm

16 Savolainen-Peltonen, H., Rahkola-Soisalo, P., Hoti, F., Vattulainen,
    P., Gissler, M., Ylikorkala, O. and Mikkola, T.S. (2019) Use of
    postmenopausal hormone therapy and risk of Alzheimer's disease in
    Finland: Nationwide case-control study. *BMJ*, 6 March, 364, l665. doi:
    10.1136/bmj.l665. PMID: 30842086; PMCID: PMC6402043.

17 (2021) Use of menopausal hormone therapy and risk of dementia:
    Nested case-control studies using QResearch and CPRD databases. *BMJ*,
    30 September, 374, n2182. doi: 10.1136/bmj.n2182

18 Pourhadi, N., Mørch, L.S., Holm, E.A., Torp-Pedersen, C. and Meaidi, A. (2023) Menopausal hormone therapy and dementia: Nationwide, nested case-control study. *BMJ*, 28 June, 381, e072770. doi: 10.1136/bmj-2022-072770. Erratum in: *BMJ*. 29 June 2023, 381, 1499. doi: 10.1136/bmj.p1499. PMID: 37380194; PMCID: PMC10302215.
19 Beam, C.R., Kaneshiro, C., Jang, J.Y., Reynolds, C.A., Pedersen, N.L. and Gatz, M. (2018) Differences between women and men in incidence rates of dementia and Alzheimer's disease. *J Alzheimers Dis*, 64(4), 1077–83. doi: 10.3233/JAD-180141. PMID: 30010124; PMCID: PMC6226313.
20 Henderson, V.W., Benke, K.S., Green, R.C., Cupples, L.A. and Farrer, L.A. (2005) MIRAGE Study Group. Postmenopausal hormone therapy and Alzheimer's disease risk: Interaction with age. *J Neurol Neurosurg Psychiatry*, January, 76(1), 103–5. doi: 10.1136/jnnp.2003.024927. PMID: 15608005; PMCID: PMC1739309.
21 Fang, M., Hu, J., Weiss, J. et al. (2025) Lifetime risk and projected burden of dementia. *Nat Med*, 13 January, doi: 10.1038/s41591-024-03340-9
22 Klijs, B., Mitratza, M., Harteloh, P., Moll van Charante, E.P., Richard, E., Nielen, M. and Kunst, A.E. (2021) Estimating the lifetime risk of dementia using nationwide individually linked cause-of-death and health register data. *International Journal of Epidemiology*, June, 50(3), 809–16, doi: 10.1093/ije/dyaa219
23 Livingston, G. et al. (2020) Dementia prevention, intervention, and care: 2020 report of The Lancet Commission. *The Lancet*, 396(10248), 413–46.
24 https://www.medicalnewstoday.com/articles/could-a-simple-eye-test-predict-alzheimers-12-years-before-symptoms-show
25 https://womensmidlifehealthjournal.biomedcentral.com/articles/10.1186/s40695-015-0002-y
26 https://www.independent.co.uk/news/health/menopause-antidepressants-symptoms-worse-hrt-shortage-a9148951.html
27 https://www.ons.gov.uk/peoplepopulationandcommunity/birthsdeathsandmarriages/deaths/bulletins/suicidesintheunitedkingdom/2023#:~:text=In%20five%2Dyear%20age%20groups,rate%20(9.2%20per%20100%2C000)
28 https://www.nice.org.uk/guidance/ng23/chapter/Recommendations
29 Thurston, R.C., Fritz, M.M., Chang, Y., Barinas Mitchell, E. and Maki, P.M. (2021) Self-compassion and subclinical cardiovascular disease among midlife women. *Health Psychol*, November 40(11), 747–53. doi: 10.1037/hea0001137. PMID: 34914480; PMCID: PMC8926023.

Chapter 8

1   Zhou, R., Guo, Q., Xiao, Y. et al. (2021) Endocrine role of bone in the regulation of energy metabolism. *Bone Res*, 9, 25. doi: 10.1038/s41413-021-00142-4

2   IMS video: 'Changing the Paradigm for Earlier Osteoporosis Prevention', https://www.youtube.com/watch?v=mNpD1F48PwU

3   Moser, S.C. and van der Erden, B.C.J. (2019) Osteocalcin: A versatile bone-derived hormone. *Endocrinol*, 10 January, 9. doi: 10.3389/fendo.2018.00794

4   Puig, J. et al. (2016) Lower serum osteocalcin concentrations are associated with brain microstructural changes and worse cognitive performance. *Clinical Endocrinology*, May, 84(5), 643–796. doi: 10.1111/cen.12954

5   Zoch, M.L., Clemens, T.L. and Riddle, R.C. (2016) New insights into the biology of osteocalcin. *Bone*, January, 82, 42–49. doi: 10.1016/j.bone.2015.05.046. Epub 6 June 2015. PMID: 26055108; PMCID: PMC4670816.

6   https://www.diabetes.co.uk/insulin/insulin-sensitivity.html

7   Moon, J.S., Jin, M.H. and Koh, H.M. (2021) Association between Serum Osteocalcin Levels and Metabolic Syndrome according to the Menopausal Status of Korean Women. *J Korean Med Sci*, 1 March, 36(8), e56. doi: 10.3346/jkms.2021.36.e56. PMID: 33650335; PMCID: PMC7921371.

8   Kanis, J. (2007) Assessment of osteoporosis at the primary health-care level. WHO Scientific Group Technical Report.

9   https://www.ncbi.nlm.nih.gov/books/NBK499878/

10 Boschitsch, E.P., Durchschlag, E., and Dimai, H.P. (2017) Age-related prevalence of osteoporosis and fragility fractures: Real-world data from an Austrian Menopause and Osteoporosis Clinic. *Climacteric*, April, 20(2): 157–63. doi: 10.1080/13697137.2017.1282452. Epub 2017 Feb 8. PMID: 28286986.

11 Varacallo, M.A., Seaman, T.J., Jandu, J.S. and Pizzutillo, P. (2023) Osteopenia. Stat Pearls. https://www.ncbi.nlm.nih.gov/books/NBK499878/

12 https://www.capturethefracture.org/policymakers#:~:text=Fragility%20Fractures%20Represent%20a%20Significant,leading%20chronic%20diseases%20%5B1%5D

13 https://www.capturethefracture.org/policymakers#:~:text=Fragility%20Fractures%20Represent%20a%20Significant,women%20%5B8%2C9%5D.

14 Morri, M., Ambrosi, E., Chiari, P. et al. (2019) One-year mortality after hip fracture surgery and prognostic factors: A prospective cohort study, *Sci Rep* 9(18718). https://doi.org/10.1038/s41598-019-55196-6

15   Watson, S.L., Weeks, B.K., Weis, L.J., Harding, A.T., Horan, S.A. and Beck, B.R. (2018) High-intensity resistance and impact training improves bone mineral density and physical function in postmenopausal women with osteopenia and osteoporosis: The LIFTMOR randomized controlled trial. *J Bone Miner Res*, February, 33(2), 211–20. doi: 10.1002/jbmr.3284. Epub 4 October 2017. Erratum in: J Bone Miner Res. 2019 March, 34(3), 572. doi: 10.1002/jbmr.3659. PMID: 28975661.

16   https://www.osteoporosis.foundation/patients/about-osteoporosis/risk-factors

17   https://theros.org.uk/information-and-support/osteoporosis/treatment/hormone-replacement-therapy/

18   Mukherjee, A. and Davis, S.R. (2025) Update on menopause hormone therapy: Current indications and unanswered questions, *Clin Endocrinol (Oxf)*, January 29. doi: 10.1111/cen.15211. Epub ahead of print. PMID: 39878309.

19   Mukherjee, A. and Davis, S.R. (2025) Update on Menopause Hormone Therapy: Current indications and unanswered questions. *Clinical Endocrinology*, 29 January. doi: 10.1111/cen.15211

20   https://www.nhs.uk/conditions/dexa-scan/

21   https://www.nhs.uk/conditions/dexa-scan/why-its-done/

22   https://www.ons.gov.uk/peoplepopulationandcommunity/healthandsocialcare/causesofdeath/articles/leadingcausesofdeathuk/2001to2018

23   Hodis, H.N. and Mack, W.J. (2022) Menopausal hormone replacement therapy and reduction of all-cause mortality and cardiovascular disease: It is about time and timing. *Cancer J*, May–Jun 01, 28(3), 208–23. doi: 10.1097/PPO.0000000000000591. PMID: 35594469; PMCID: PMC9178928.

24   Rodgers, J.L., Jones, J., Bolleddu, S.I., Vanthenapalli, S., Rodgers, L.E., Shah, K., Karia, K. and Panguluri, S.K. (2019) Cardiovascular risks associated with gender and aging. *J Cardiovasc Dev Dis*, April, 6(2), 19. doi: 10.3390/jcdd6020019. PMID: 31035613; PMCID: PMC6616540. https://pmc.ncbi.nlm.nih.gov/articles/PMC6616540/

25   https://www.health.harvard.edu/heart-health/the-heart-disease-gender-gap

26   https://www.escardio.org/The-ESC/Press-Office/Press-releases/Women-more-likely-to-die-after-heart-attack-than-men#:~:text=At%20five%20years%2C%20one%2Dthird,close%20the%20gap%20in%20outcomes.%E2%80%9D

27   Devlon, H.A., Mirzaei and S. Zegre-Hemsey, J. (2020) Typical and Atypical Symptoms of Acute Coronary Syndrome: Time to Retire the

Terms? *Journal of the American Heart Association*, 25 March, 9(7). doi: 10.11T61/JAHA.119.015539.PMID: 32208828

28 https://www.bhf.org.uk/informationsupport/heart-matters-magazine/medical/ask-the-experts/are-heart-attack-symptoms-different-for-men-and-women

29 Parlati, A. L. M., Nardi, E., Sucato, V., Madaudo, C., Leo, G., Rajah, T., Marzano, F., Prastaro, M., Gargiulo, P., Paolillo, S., Vadalà, G., Galassi, A. R., Perrone Filardi, P. (2025) ANOCA, INOCA, MINOCA: The New frontier of coronary syndromes. *J. Cardiovasc Dev Dis*, February 10; 12(2): 64. doi: 10.3390/jcdd12020064. PMID: 39997498; PMCID: PMC11856364.

30 Schamroth Pravda, N., Karny-Rahkovich, O., Shiyovich, A., Schamroth Pravda, M., Rapeport, N., Vaknin-Assa, H., Eisen, A., Kornowski, R. and Porter, A. (2021) Coronary artery disease in women: A comprehensive appraisal. *J Clin Med*, 12 October, 10(20), 4664. doi: 10.3390/jcm10204664. PMID: 34682787; PMCID: PMC8541551.

31 https://www.heart.org/en/news/2018/07/13/uncommon-heart-attack-found-more-often-in-women-needs-a-second-look

32 https://www.health.harvard.edu/heart-health/the-heart-disease-gender-gap

33 Sattar, Y., Siew, K.S.W., Connerney, M., Ullah, W. and Alraies, M.C. (2020) Management of Takotsubo Syndrome: A Comprehensive Review. *Cureus*, 3 January, 12(1), e6556. doi: 10.7759/cureus.6556. PMID: 32042529; PMCID: PMC6996473.

34 https://www.acc.org/About-ACC/Press-Releases/2024/04/01/21/39/heart-health-declines-rapidly-after-menopause

35 Roeters van Lennep, J.E. et al. (2023) Women, lipids, and atherosclerotic cardiovascular disease: A call to action from the European Atherosclerosis Society. *European Heart Journal*, October, 44(39), 4157–73. doi: 10.1093/eurheartj/ehad472

Chapter 9

1 https://d3nkl3psvxxpe9.cloudfront.net/documents/YG-Archive-WomensBodiesInternal-070219.pdf

2 https://www.buzzfeed.com/erinlarosa/how-many-words-that-mean-vagina-do-you-know

3 https://www.womanandhome.com/life/news-entertainment/Gillian-Anderson-yoni-dress-embroidery/

4 https://finance.yahoo.com/news/women-intimate-care-product-market-103000472.html

5 Carlson, K. and Nguyen, H. (2025) Genitourinary Syndrome of Menopause. StatPearls. https://www.ncbi.nlm.nih.gov/books/NBK559297/

6   Genitourinary Syndrome of Menopause. https://www.ncbi.nlm.nih.
    gov/books/NBK559297/#:~:text=GSM%20impacts%2027%25%20to%20
    84,stimulation%20of%20the%20urogenital%20tissues
7   Meaidi, A., Pourhadi, N., Løkkegaard, E.C., Torp-Pedersen, C. and
    Steinrud Mørch, L. (2024) Association of vaginal oestradiol and the rate
    of breast cancer in Denmark: Registry based, case-control study, nested
    in a nationwide cohort. *BMJ Medicine*, 3, e000753.
8   https://www.bgcs.org.uk/wp-content/uploads/2024/09/BGCS-BMS-
    Guidelines-on-Management-of-Menopausal-Symptoms-after-
    Gynaecological-Cancer-09.09.24.pdf
9   Palacios, S. (2020) Expression of androgen receptors in the structures
    of vulvovaginal tissue. *Menopause*, November, 27(11): 1336–42. doi:
    10.1097/GME.0000000000001587. PMID: 33110052.
10 Thomas, H.M., Bryce, C.L., Ness, R.B. and Hess, R. (2011) Dyspareunia
    is associated with decreased frequency of intercourse in the menopausal
    transition. *Menopause*, February, 18(2), 152–57. doi: 10.1097/
    gme.0b013e3181eeb774. PMID: 20962696; PMCID: PMC3026887.
11 Rubin, R. (2023) Vaginal dryness can be fatal. No, really. Medscape,
    11 October. https://www.medscape.com/viewarticle/996829
12 Overview of Outcomes for Inpatient Stays Involving Sepsis, 2016–2021.
    https://hcup-us.ahrq.gov/reports/statbriefs/sb306-overview-sepsis-
    2016-2021.pdf
13 https://sepsistrust.org/wp-content/uploads/2024/11/YHEC-Sepsis-
    Report-17.02.17-FINAL.pdf
14 https://researchbriefings.files.parliament.uk/documents/CDP-2024-
    0122/CDP-2024-0122.pdf
15 Wood, K.A. and Angus, D.C. (2004) Pharmacoeconomic implications
    of new therapies. *Pharmacoeconomics*, 22(14), 895–906. doi: 10.2165/
    00019053-200422140-00001. PMID: 15362927.
16 Eriksson, I., Gustafson, Y., Fagerström, L. and Olofsson, B. (2010)
    Prevalence and factors associated with urinary tract infections (UTIs) in
    very old women. *Arch Gerontol Geriatr*, March–April, 50(2), 132–35. doi:
    10.1016/j.archger.2009.02.013. Epub 5 April 2009. PMID: 19349084.
17 https://www.england.nhs.uk/wp-content/uploads/2015/08/Sepsis-
    Action-Plan-23.12.15-v1.pdf
18 Wagenlehner, F. et al. (2013) Diagnosis and management for urosepsis.
    Int J Urol, October, 20(10), 963–70. doi: 10.1111/iju.12200. Epub 29 May
    2013.
19 Mark, K.P., Arenella, K. Girard, A., Herbenick, D., Fu, J. and Coleman, E.
    (2024) Erectile dysfunction prevalence in the United States: Report from
    the 2021 National Survey of Sexual Wellbeing. *The Journal of Sexual
    Medicine*, 26 February, 21(4), 296–303, doi: 10.1093/jsxmed/qdae008

20 Tan-Kim, J., Sha, N.M., Do, D. and Menefee, S.A. (2023) Efficacy of vaginal estrogen for recurrent urinary tract infection prevention in hypoestrogenic women. *Am J Obstet Gynecol*, August, 229(2), 143, e1–143, e9. doi: 10.1016/j.ajog.2023.05.002

21 https://www.nice.org.uk/guidance/ng112/chapter/Recommendations#treatments-for-preventing-recurrent-uti

22 Rowe, T.A. and Juthani-Mehta, M. (2013) Urinary tract infection in older adults. *Aging Health*, October, 9(5): 10. doi: 10.2217/ahe.13.38. PMID: 24391677; PMCID: PMC3878051.

23 https://www.england.nhs.uk/south/2023/10/12/older-people-across-the-south-west-urged-to-protect-themselves-against-urinary-tract-infections/#:~:text=UTIs%20can%20be%20particularly%20serious,for%20people%20aged%2095%2Dplus

24 Thomas-White, K., Taege, S., Limeira, R., Brincat, C., Joyce, C., Hilt, E.E., Mac-Daniel, L., Radek, K.A., Brubaker, L., Mueller, E.R. and Wolfe, A.J. (2020) Vaginal estrogen therapy is associated with increased Lactobacillus in the urine of postmenopausal women with overactive bladder symptoms. *Am J Obstet Gynecol*, November, 223(5), 727, e1–727.e11. doi: 10.1016/j.ajog.2020.08.006. Epub 11 August 2020. PMID: 32791124; PMCID: PMC7609597.

25 Cody, J.D., Jacobs, M.L., Richardson, K., Moehrer, B. and Hextall, A. (2012) Oestrogen therapy for urinary incontinence in post-menopausal women. *Cochrane Database Syst Rev*, 17 October, 10(10), CD001405. doi: 10.1002/14651858.CD001405.pub3. PMID: 23076892; PMCID: PMC7086391.

26 https://iris.who.int/bitstream/handle/10665/76580/WHO_RHR_12.33_eng.pdf

27 Edwards, D. and Panay, N. (2016) Treating vulvovaginal atrophy/genitourinary syndrome of menopause: How important is vaginal lubricant and moisturizer composition? *Climacteric*, April, 19(2): 151–61. doi: 10.3109/13697137.2015.1124259. Epub December 26 2015. PMID: 26707589; PMCID: PMC4819835.

Chapter 10

1 https://www.sleepfoundation.org/women-sleep/menopause-and-sleep

2 https://www.hopkinsmedicine.org/health/wellness-and-prevention/how-does-menopause-affect-my-sleep

3 https://www.hopkinsmedicine.org/health/wellness-and-prevention/how-does-menopause-affect-my-sleep

4 Jessen, N.A., Munk, A.S., Lundgaard, I. and Nedergaard, M. (2015) The glymphatic system: A beginner's guide. *Neurochem Res*, December,

40(12), 2583–99. doi: 10.1007/s11064-015-1581-6. Epub 7 May 2015. PMID: 25947369; PMCID: PMC4636982.

5   Carson, M.Y. and Thurston, R.C. (2023) Vasomotor symptoms and their links to cardiovascular disease risk. *Curr Opin Endocr Metab Res*, Jun, 30, 100448. doi: 10.1016/j.coemr.2023.100448. Epub 18 April 2023. PMID: 37214424; PMCID: PMC10198127.

6   Jehan, S., Auguste, E., Zizi, F., Pandi-Perumal, S.R., Gupta, R., Attarian, H., Jean-Louis, G. and McFarlane, S.I. (2016) Obstructive sleep apnea: Women's perspective. *J Sleep Med Disord*, 3(6), 1064. Epub 25 August 2016. PMID: 28239685; PMCID: PMC5323064.

7   https://www.mayoclinic.org/diseases-conditions/sleep-apnea/diagnosis-treatment/drc-20377636

8   https://www.nhs.uk/conditions/sleep-apnoea/

9   https://www.thensf.org/do-i-have-insomnia/#:~:text=Look%20Out%20for%20These%20Symptoms&text=Insomnia%20symptoms%20vary%20from%20person,long%20periods%20during%20the%20night

10   https://www.sleepfoundation.org/insomnia/treatment/cognitive-behavioral-therapy-insomnia

11   https://www.thensf.org/sleep-health-topics/

12   Doherty, R., Madigan, S., Nevill, A., Warrington, G. and Ellis, J.G. (2023) The impact of kiwifruit consumption on the sleep and recovery of elite athletes. *Nutrients*, 11 May, 15(10), 2274. doi: 10.3390/nu15102274. PMID: 37242157; PMCID: PMC10220871.

13   https://www.aad.org/public/everyday-care/skin-care-secrets/anti-aging/skin-care-during-menopause

14   Liang, S.Y. (2016) Sepsis and other infectious disease emergencies in the elderly. *Emerg Med Clin North Am*, August, 34(3), 501–22. doi: 10.1016/j.emc.2016.04.005. PMID: 27475012; PMCID: PMC5022369.

15   Passos-Soares, J.S. et al. (2017) Association between osteoporosis treatment and severe periodontitis in postmenopausal women. *Menopause*, February. https://journals.lww.com/menopausejournal/Abstract/2017/07000/Association_between_osteoporosis_treatment_and.12.aspx

16   Morimoto, T., Hirata, H., Sugita, K., Paholpak, P., Kobayashi, T., Tanaka, T., Kato, K., Tsukamoto, M., Umeki, S., Toda, Y. and Mawatari, M. (2024) A view on the skin-bone axis: Unraveling similarities and potential of crosstalk. *Front Med (Lausanne)*, 4 March, 11, 1360483. doi: 10.3389/fmed.2024.1360483. PMID: 38500951; PMCID: PMC10944977.

17   https://www.bhf.org.uk/informationsupport/heart-matters-magazine/research/gum-disease-heart-health#:~:text=If%20left%20untreated%2C%20this%20can,heart%20or%20blood%20vessel%20problems

18 Pan, M.Y., Hsieh, T.C., Chen, P.H. and Chen, M.Y. (2019) Factors associated with tooth loss in postmenopausal women: A community-based cross-sectional study. *Int J Environ Res Public Health*, 16 October, 16(20), 3945. doi: 10.3390/ijerph16203945. PMID: 31623275; PMCID: PMC6843320.

19 https://www.medscape.com/viewarticle/regular-flossing-tied-reduced-ischemic-stroke-risk-2025a10002t7

20 https://www.nidcr.nih.gov/health-info/dry-mouth#helpful-tips

21 Vonda, J., Wright, J.D., Schwartzman, R.I. and Wittstein, J. (2024) The musculoskeletal syndrome of menopause. *Climacteric*, 27(5), 466–472, doi: 10.1080/13697137.2024.2380363

Chapter 11

1 https://www.statista.com/statistics/870238/proportion-of-women-in-uk-cabinets/

2 https://www.msci.com/research-and-insights/women-on-boards-and-beyond-2023#:~:text=Women%20held%2025.8%25%20of%20board,more%20than%20doubled%20since%202019

3 https://www.mckinsey.com/featured-insights/diversity-and-inclusion/diversity-wins-how-inclusion-matters

4 https://www.hrmagazine.co.uk/content/news/childcare-costs-forcing-mothers-to-quit-work/

5 https://www.hse.gov.uk/mothers/employer/workplace-safety-law.htm#:~:text=The%20Equality%20Act%202010%20makes,new%20mother%20or%20are%20breastfeeding

6 Steffan, B. and Loretto, W. (2024) Menopause, work and mid-life: Challenging the ideal worker stereotype. *Gender Work & Organization*, 32(3), doi: 10.1111/gwao.13136

7 https://www.equalityhumanrights.com/equality-watchdog-supports-important-tribunal-hearing-alleged-menopause-discrimination

8 https://www.lodders.co.uk/direct-line-tribunal-determines-menopause-a-disability/#:~:text=In%20a%20recent%20tribunal%2C%20a,reasonable%20adjustments%20for%20her%20symptoms

9 https://www.thetimes.com/uk/article/menopause-disability-employers-work-s33cct5b6

10 https://www.equalityhumanrights.com/guidance/menopause-workplace-guidance-employers

11 https://academic.oup.com/heapro/article/39/6/daae150/7906022

12 https://www.dearmenopause.au/95-behind-the-scenes-of-australias-menopause-movement-with-johanna-wicks/

13 https://www.theguardian.com/society/2025/feb/26/a-landmark-australian-inquiry-put-the-spotlight-on-menopause-but-was-the-process-transparent-ntwnfb
14 https://publications.parliament.uk/pa/cm/cmallparty/220907/menopause.htm
15 https://publications.parliament.uk/pa/cm/cmallparty/231101/menopause.htm
16 https://publications.parliament.uk/pa/cm/cmallparty/230111/menopause.htm
17 Gentilini, A. and Parvanova, I. (2023) Industry funding of patient organisations in the UK: A retrospective study of commercial determinants, funding concentration and disease prevalence. *BMJ Open*, 13, e071138. doi: 10.1136/bmjopen-2022-071138
18 Holman, B., Geislar, S. (2018) Sex drugs and corporate ventriloquism: How to evaluate science policies intended to manage industry-funded bias. *Philosophy of Science*, 85(5): 869–81. doi:10.1086/69971319 https://menopause.org/wp-content/uploads/professional/2023-nonhormone-therapy-position-statement.pdf
20 Hansard. https://hansard.parliament.uk/commons/2022-06-09/debates/5EEB4A70-CDA6-4474-B440-3CF855FD4713/Menopause

Chapter 12

1 https://news.uga.edu/evolutionary-purpose-menopause-research/#:~:text=It%20was%20also%20referred%20to,the%20laboratory%2C%20and%20by%201938
2 https://www.gsb.stanford.edu/faculty-research/publications/intersectional-escape-older-women-elude-agentic-prescriptions-more
3 https://www.guidantfinancial.com/small-business-trends/2024-women-in-business/
4 https://www.ucl.ac.uk/news/2024/jan/cold-water-swimming-improves-menopause-symptoms#:~:text=Menopausal%20women%20who%20regularly%20swim,athletes'%20muscle%20repair%20and%20recovery
5 https://www.cdc.gov/womens-health/lcod/females.html
6 https://thebms.org.uk/wp-content/uploads/2023/01/WHC-Infographics-JANUARY-2023-BreastCancerRisks.pdf
7 https://www.goodreads.com/quotes/11923487-it-is-a-well-known-fact-and-one-that-has-given

Acknowledgements

Over the past few years, I've had the privilege to meet some amazing, passionate and dedicated people who are working incredibly hard, some for absolutely nothing in monetary terms, to change the future of women's health. They come from a diverse set of professions and backgrounds: grassroots campaigners, the fitness industry, the medical and allied health, policy and politics, and the media. I'm not going to name them all because I know I'll forget someone, and I don't want to leave anyone out.

I've also had the privilege of virtually connecting with thousands of women and listening to their sometimes harrowing stories as they've made their way through this period. And to those of you who have trusted me with your stories and experiences – a big hug and thank you. In many ways this book is for you.

For the book itself I cannot thank enough the pool of exceptionally talented and caring people who have given me access to their brains! I thank each and every one of them for their time and contribution. In particular, and in alphabetical order: Drs Reem Al-Shaikh, Juliet Balfour, Sam Brown, Elise Dallas, Itunu Johnson-Sogbetun, Mandy Leonhardt, Ginni Mansberg, Louise Newson, Naomi Potter (who did her first ever Instagram live with me – and look at her now!), Aziza Sesay and Carys Sonnenberg, and menopause expert and pharmacist Kate Organ, endocrinologists Professors Susan Davis and Annice Muhkerjee, reproductive health specialist Joyce Harper and gynaecologists Michelle Griffin, Mary Claire Haver MD, Pauline Maki (PhD as well as professor of psychiatry and psychology), Shilpa McQuillan, Janice Rymer and Lauren Streicher MD, consultant dermatologists Claire Kiely and Angela Tewari, and professor of psychiatry Jayashri Kulkarni. On the diet side – a big thank you too to the very trustworthy, no-nonsense dietician Elizabeth Ward.

In the non-medical arena, a huge thanks as well to big brains across the world like advocate, lawyer and policy expert Jennifer Weiss-Wolf in New York, academics Dr Josie Hamper and Hannah Swift here in the UK, and Ray Moynihan and Professor Samantha Thomas in Australia, all of whom gave me their time and insights. A big thank you too to the wonderful Sam Evans for her 'sexpertise' and Cathy Procter, Kate Oakey, Madhu Kapoor and Vicky Shattock for sharing their personal experiences, all of whom have been in this space supporting people for such a long time.

Then there are those who took the time to read bits and give me constructive feedback – the amazing health editor Lynnette Hoffman (we've worked together for more than 20 years but have never physically met!), Racheal Edgerton, Kirsten Sittard, Drs Alison MacBeth and Zoe Hodson, and my old university friend Irene Thompson. Much appreciated! Special shout out to Mandy Leonhardt here again for her eagle eye on fact checking and Dr Jungwoo Kang and Dan Haxby for checking my maths.

And, to my partners at the Menopause Research and Education Fund, not just trustees but my trusty brains trust – the wonderful and generous people, Associate Professor Vikram Talaulikar and Diane Danzebrink, both of whom have tirelessly campaigned for menopausal women for many years. A mega thank you to both of you for all you do, your reliability, level heads, depth of knowledge and commitment to making the world a better place.

And, of course, my patient publisher Victoria Roddam and her team – who gave me just ten weeks to write this, but at least had the (possibly misplaced) faith that I could put out something vaguely researched and coherent in such a short time.

And last but not least, my family. My husband who made me lunch each day, listened patiently when I threw ideas at him, and took Maddie (our giant and very loud German Shepherd) away so I could at least have a couple of hours each day without her barking and causing me to jump about a metre into the air and forget what I was just about to type. And my son and daughter-in-law who have sat for years through dinners with their eyes glazing over as I've prattled on about menopause, vaginas and health inequities. Unfortunately, that's probably not going to stop!

Thank you and big love to you all!

Index